Body & Beauty Care

Dr. Neena Khanna, MBBS, MD
Additional Professor
All India Institute of Medical Sciences, New Delhi

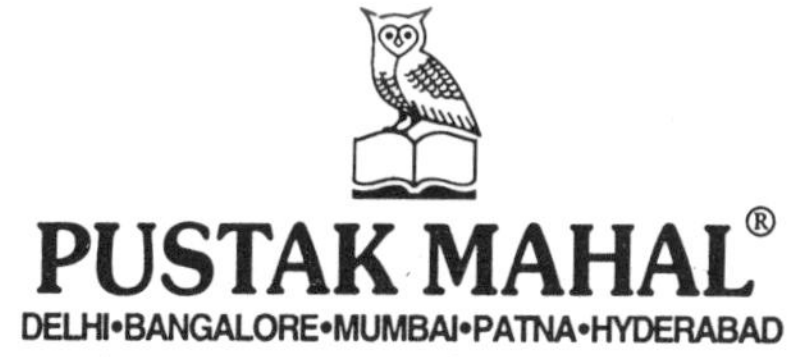

PUSTAK MAHAL®
DELHI•BANGALORE•MUMBAI•PATNA•HYDERABAD

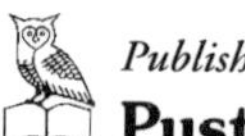
Publishers
Pustak Mahal®
J-3/16 , Daryaganj, New Delhi-110002
☎ 23276539, 23272783, 23272784 • *Fax:* 011-23260518
E-mail: info@pustakmahal.com • *Website:* www.pustakmahal.com

Sales Centre
- 10-B, Netaji Subhash Marg, Daryaganj, New Delhi-110002
  ☎ 23268292, 23268293, 23279900 • *Fax:* 011-23280567
  E-mail: rapidexdelhi@indiatimes.com
- **Hind Pustak Bhawan**
  6686, Khari Baoli, Delhi-110006
  ☎ 23944314, 23911979

Branches
Bengaluru: ☎ 080-22234025 • *Telefax:* 080-22240209
E-mail: pustak@airtelmail.in • pustak@sancharnet.in
Mumbai: ☎ 022-22010941, 022-22053387
E-mail: rapidex@bom5.vsnl.net.in
Patna: ☎ 0612-3294193 • *Telefax:* 0612-2302719
E-mail: rapidexptn@rediffmail.com
Hyderabad: *Telefax:* 040-24737290
E-mail: pustakmahalhyd@yahoo.co.in

ISBN 978-81-223-0098-7

Edition: 2011

Printed at : Unique Colour Cartoon, Delhi

PREFACE

The image a person projects is of basic and significant importance in career development, opportunity, peer status and ultimate achievement. It has often been thought that well-groomed persons are generally more sensitive, kind, interesting, strong, poised, sociable, outgoing and exciting than poorly groomed individuals.

The importance of beauty has long been appreciated by poets and artists. Today much can be done with cosmetics to enhance the appearance of an individual. Cosmetics contribute not only to the appearance but also to health in the fullest sense of psychological and social wholesomeness.

This book is primarily intended for the new conscious generation of men and women who groom to look good. It is for those people who want to scientifically appear fabulous and want to know what they are using to look glamorous. The book will help you in differentiating between what is the right way and the wrong way of doing things.

Starting with a basic knowledge of the structures and functioning of skin, nail, hair and teeth, the book goes on to cover normal care of parts of the body which are 'on show'. Various myths have been dispelled scientifically and the book does not subscribe to the effect of unscientific instant remedies. One objective of this book is to give information concerning the major categories of cosmetic products with emphasis on intended uses, generalities of formulations and an update on what is new. This I feel is very important because most women are totally confused by the vast range of cosmetic products available.

Another objective is to review specific problems caused by cosmetics. Use of correct cosmetic products for people with different skin types and how each cosmetic category can be used to the fullest advantage is discussed in great detail.

A part of the book is devoted to the cause and effect of common skin, hair, nail and teeth problems. It provides sound practical advice on the treatment of these problems. A separate chapter deals with the modern trends in cosmetic surgery – a field which is attracting a lot of clientele today. However, readers are strictly advised to seek expert medical opinion and not indulge in self treatment.

—Neena Khanna

ACKNOWLEDGEMENTS

Three great teachers have played a very dominant role in shaping my career as a dermatologist. Prof R.K. Pandhi has been my guide and confidant for several years. He was the one who initiated me into writing this book – *Body and Beauty Care.* Prof L.K. Bhutani has been my teacher and advisor and has helped me through many a crisis. Prof J.S. Pasricha has constantly encouraged me to write effectively. This book is, in a sense, tribute to my three teachers, even though the book does not deal purely with dermatology.

There are several sections of this book which would not have been complete without the help of several of my colleagues and friends. Ms Chandralekha Patel, a renowned cosmetologist gave me valuable suggestions and helped me immensely to compile the section on 'Application of Makeup'. Dr Ritu Duggal and Ms Jasbir Kaur helped and critically evaluated the sections on 'Teeth Care' and 'Weight Problems' respectively. Ms Neera Saldhana, a physiotherapist, gave me extremely useful suggestions on the exercises incorporated in the book.

Ms Felci rendered not only outstanding and timely secretarial assistance but also helped me tremendously with the editing of the manuscript.

I would like to thank my parents, who were a constant and an unfailing source of encouragement and inspiration and this book would just not have been possible without their help and support.

Last but not the least, my appreciation for all the assistance to Anil, who helped me to finish this work despite all odds.

CONTENTS

1. Skin and Skin Care

We all begin our lives with a soft and smooth skin, but not many of us can boast of a finely textured skin by the time we are thirty. This is because most of us take our skin, the largest organ in the body, very much for granted. Remember, your skin can get tired if not looked after, and that it, like any other living tissue, really does respond to tender care and attention. If you realise how full of life your skin is and understand how it performs its various functions, skin-care will become at once more logical and more easily undertaken. Understanding your skin will also enable you to make an active use of your skin in relating more positively to your environment and in communicating with your fellow human beings.

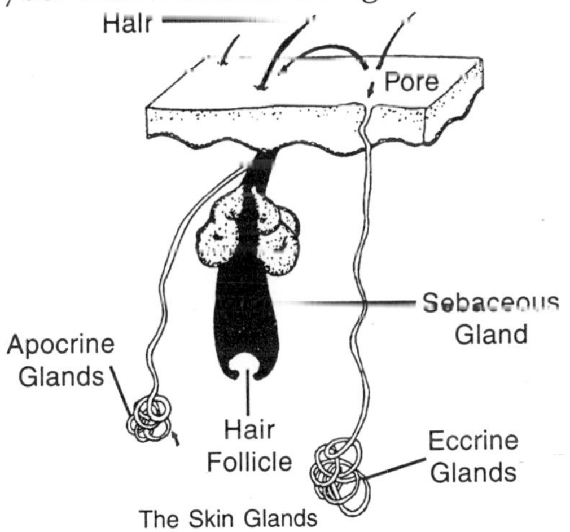

Fig. 1. Your skin under the microscope.

STRUCTURE AND FUNCTION OF YOUR SKIN

Skin consists of three layers — the epidermis, the dermis, and the subcutaneous tissue. The surface epidermis is a relatively thin layer. Beneath the epidermis is the thicker and the much stronger dermis. The subcutaneous tissue or the fat containing layer lies below the dermis. (Fig. 1).

The epidermis

The epidermis is a fairly thin layer. Its thickness varies around the body, depending on the special needs of that area. For instance, the epidermis over the eyelids is particularly thin, while that over the palms and soles is very thick.

The epidermis is itself made up of several layers. On the surface is the horny layer — the *stratum corneum*. This layer is made up of dead cells, which are continuously being shed. The cells are shed off as small aggregates which are normally too small to be seen; sometimes, however, these aggregates become larger and are then visible as scales. This is exactly what happens in dandruff or when our skin is deprived of moisture.

Below the layer of dead cells are stacks of living cells comprising the *stratum malpighi*. This layer produces the main skin protein known as *Keratin*. The lowermost layer of the epidermis or the basal layer is where new cells are produced. These new cells take about a month to travel to the surface. In some diseases, however, the movement of the cells to the surface is speeded up and this results in scaling.

The skin pigment, *melanin*, is produced by special cells called melanocytes. Melanin is very important for the protection of the skin from the sun; this is precisely the reason why melanocytes are stimulated on exposure to the sun, resulting in darkening of the skin.

The dermis

The dermis is a much thicker layer than the epidermis. It is made up of a connective tissue framework in which are embedded blood vessels, lymph vessels, nerves, several types of glands, hair and a whole variety of cells. The connective tissue of the dermis is predominantly made up of a protein called *collagen*. Presently, this protein is being popularly used for the treatment of a variety of skin problems like wrinkles and scars. I will talk about it in greater detail in a later chapter. *Elastin* or elastic fibres are the other type of protein fibres in the dermis.

The dermis also contains a complex system of blood and lymph vessels and a highly complicated nervous system. The nerves receive and pass on an endless stream of valuable information to the body. Any type of skin massage is thought to facilitate the drainage of lymph glands and also to enhance the circulation of blood. Similarly, it has been suggested that massages soothe the nerves in the skin.

The subcutaneous tissue

Below the dermis is the fat storage bank of the skin. The amount of the fat stored varies in different parts of the body. In some parts of the body it has been given fancy names like '*cellulite*'. This tissue has been a source of considerable controversy in scientific and cosmetic circles.

The skin glands

The dermis has three types of glands: the apocrine glands, the eccrine sweat glands, and the sebaceous glands.

The *sebaceous glands* are present throughout the entire surface of the skin, except the palms and soles. They are particularly numerous in the scalp and on the face. These glands open into the hair follicles and secrete an oily lubricant — the sebum. This contains cholesterol, fatty acids and waxes. Sebum forms a thin film which lubricates the skin; it also forms a coating on the hair, keeping them soft and shiny. When sebaceous secretions are inadequate, the epidermis becomes dry and wrinkled and when the glands secrete heavily, the skin becomes oily and shiny. These glands are involved in acne (pimples).

The *apocrine glands* are present in association with the hair follicles. They are found mainly in areas where there is obvious body hair such as in the armpits and around the genital area. These glands are under hormonal control. A large part of the body odour can be traced to the apocrine glands. By themselves, the secretions of these glands are odourless, but bacteria (which are normally present on the skin) act on the secretions to produce the characteristic body odour.

The *eccrine sweat glands* are distributed widely over the skin and produce a much larger amount of secretions. These glands are concerned with the regulation of body temperature. Under normal circumstances, the sweat glands produce about half a litre of sweat in a day. In very hot climates, the generation of sweat is increased tremendously and as the water is lost, the body cools down.

Functions of the skin

The functions of the skin are truly a paradox — skin is both a barrier surrounding and protecting your body from innumerable external assaults and at the same time, it is the means of your constant contact with the environment. One of its main jobs is to regulate temperature. Another is to prevent germs and poisons from invading the body. Just as important is its task of preventing the loss of body fluids, as it forms an almost waterproof barrier. Simultaneously, it also functions as an active organ of excretion, helping to rid the body of wastes in the form of sweat.

On a psychological level, your skin is the most active link with your surroundings. Quite apart from its role in your personal appearance, the skin is vital in conveying the sense of touch and forms the principal organ of sexual attraction and communication.

Skin types

It is really very important for you to be able to identify your skin type. This is to enable you to look after your skin correctly. Also the selection of your cosmetics is, to a considerable extent, influenced by your skin type. Although no two skins are exactly similar most have characteristics which enable them to be grouped into one of the following types: normal skin, dry skin, oily skin, and combination skin.

Normal skin: This skin is smooth and velvety to touch and does not look puffy or shiny. The skin has a rosy colour because the circulation of blood is good and the skin is well moisturised. The pores are fine and barely visible. This type of skin is something of a rarity. If you own this type of skin, you have a real fortune to exploit. However, though, this type of skin is not really problematic, it still needs sensible care and gentle treatment. Choose your skin care products carefully and always look for mild, well-balanced cosmetics.

Dry skin: This skin is fine, delicate and dry with a tendency to scaling on the cheeks. Underneath, the skin lacks suppleness and therefore feels taut after washing. The pores are not visible as there is an insufficient amount of secretion from the sebaceous glands. Dry skin tends to age prematurely and is wrinkle-prone unless nurtured. Constant protection is very important and the products used must be gentle, rich and soothing. Always use a moisturizer during the day and a good cream at night.

Oily skin: This skin is coarse, thick and shiny. The sebaceous glands being over-active, the pores are clearly visible. Oily skin is prone to comedones (white heads and black heads) and pimples and needs to be cleaned scrupulously. Only those cosmetics which have been formulated especially for oily skins should be used, otherwise there will be problems.

Combination skin: Most of us have a combination skin. The middle of the face (patches on the forehead, the nose and the chin) is shiny with dilated ostia and a coarse texture (Fig.2). The rest of the face is either normal or dry. Sometimes, the difference between the two areas is great; if such is the case with your skin, then you would have to treat each part of the face accordingly — the dry areas as for dry skin and the central panel as for oily skin.

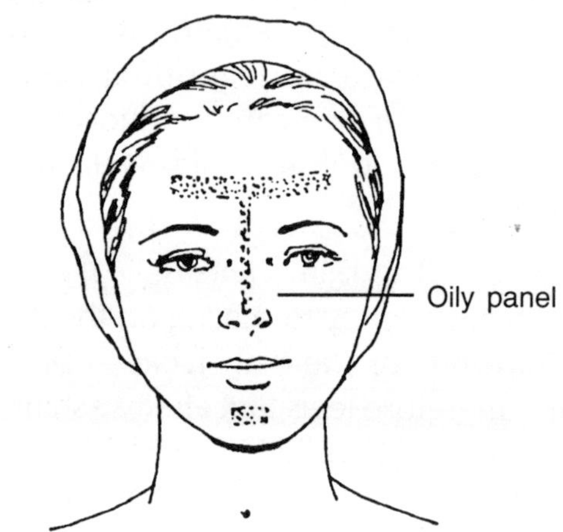

Fig. 2. The oily panel of the combination skin.

pH of the skin

For decades, cosmetic manufacturers have done considerable research in order to discover and produce products whose pH is healthiest for the skin and the hair. The symbol pH is used in everyday language to represent the degree of acidity or alkalinity of a substance. When a solution is neither alkaline nor acidic, it is called neutral. For example, the pH of pure water, a neutral substance, is 7. If the pH of a solution is less than 7, it is acidic; if the pH is greater than 7, it is alkaline.

The pH of healthy normal skin is between 5.2 and 6; i.e., it is slightly acidic. This acidic pH of the skin is due to the presence of acids in the sebum, sweat, and keratin. It is necessary to maintain the acidity of the skin. This is, probably, the reason why it is thought that curds and lemon juice when applied would do wonders for your skin. This is also the reason why ordinary soaps (which are alkaline) have, rather erroneously, got themselves a bad name.

DIET AND YOUR SKIN

Diet and your skin

If you want a healthy skin, it is important for you to have a healthy diet — a diet which contains adequate amounts of vitamins, minerals and proteins. Balance is the key word. No single diet is responsible for building up or maintaining the skin — so fad diets, which over-emphasise one food in preference to others can actually deprive you of essential nutrients and so may even harm your body and skin.

Moreover, there are a lot of misconceptions about the effect of certain foods on your skin. It is not true, for instance, that eating chocolates, sweets or rich cakes will give you spots (your waistline may, however widen!). Neither is it true that eating greasy, fried foods will give you a greasy skin or make your hair greasy. Nor can it be guaranteed, that if you fill yourself up with cucumbers, grapes, carrot juice or lettuce you will acquire a beautiful, flawless complexion. Some people have even come out with extraordinary claims, suggesting, for example, that salads will dramatically change your appearance and to develop a perfect skin you must take vitamin and mineral supplements. All this to my mind is humbug. Although there is no denying that you must take a varied and a balanced diet, it is equally important to remember that the single most important factor in determining the beauty of your complexion is heredity and that your eating habits play only a very small part in it.

However, if your diet is grossly deficient in certain elements, then the skin can develop problems. In people taking normal balanced diets this does not happen. But after severe illness, surgery and in people who are on crash diets, problems might occur.

With gross nutritional deficiencies, as occurs in severe illness of any type, the skin becomes dry and dark. The lips become sore, the hair falls, and the nails develop ridges and may even get discoloured. The feet become swollen.

Vitamin A is very important for the health of your skin and eyes. The richest sources of this vitamin are cod-liver oil, liver, carrots, spinach, milk, and egg-yolk. If the diet is lacking in this vitamin, the skin becomes excessively dry and develops pimples. Vision at night becomes defective. But remember, neither should you overdose yourself with Vitamin A, because this also can cause dryness and roughness of the skin, falling of the hair and soreness of lips. Cracking and soreness of lips also develop in vitamin B deficiencies. Liver, meat, milk, greens, pulses and cereals are rich sources of vitamin B. Vitamin C, found in all citrus fruits (lemons, oranges etc.), is also needed for the health of your skin. Vitamin E has been touted as panacea for several ills of the skin — this may well be an exaggeration. There is no denying that vitamin E is an antioxidant and reduces photodamage (damage of the skin when exposed to sun), both when taken orally and applied locally. It, however, has very little effect on stretch marks and sometimes, when incorporated in cosmetics, can actually cause allergic reactions.

Apart from vitamins, your diet should also include minerals. Iron makes the blood healthy — consequently it imparts a healthy pink glow to your skin. Iron is found in several green vegetables, in fruits and in meats. Zinc is also very important for the health of your skin.

Beverages and skin

Many beverages can actually harm the skin. Alcohol and coffee cause the small blood vessels, under the skin surface to widen. This results in the familiar flushed look. Though, the effects of both alcohol and coffee are initially only temporary, excessive drinking will cause permanent widening of blood vessels making them apparent as thread veins. There are also several other causes of thread veins:

heredity, effects of the sun, a highly spiced diet and extremes of temperature. You can't help inheriting your genes, but you can certainly avoid the other factors to retard the appearance of thread veins.

Is tea healthy?

Tea is naturally relaxing and refreshing. This unassuming brew has become one of the hottest ingredients of natural cosmetics today. Tea is a strong antioxidant rich in vitamin C and E. It is a powerful enemy of free radicals that cause aging. The polyphenols in tea fight plaque causing dental bacteria. It is a rich source of fluoride and fights tooth decay. Tea contains flavonoids which help fight heart disease. Tea contains essential minerals and vitamins. (I am not saying all this because I guzzle down several cups of tea!) However, remember not to drink tea with your meals because tea may decrease absorption of iron and this may result in anaemia.

Food allergies and skin problems

Foods often play an important role in causing, at least, two types of skin problems – hives and eczemas. Though, there are several types of eczemas which are not due to food allergies, 'atopic eczema' is often worsened by certain food items such as milk, eggs and preserved foods. A person may also be allergic to more than one food stuff. Often a number of hours elapse before the skin reaction occurs; so it is quite a problem to identify the culprit. Luckily, most people outgrow their food allergies and it is really not always necessary to search very carefully for the causative agent.

SKIN AND YOUR ENVIRONMENT

Natural moisture in the skin

The moisture content of the skin really means its water content – this is the most important factor which governs its softness and elasticity and is responsible for its youthful appearance. But water is constantly being lost from the skin surface (apart from what is lost through sweating) and this loss is continuously being replaced from below. There are two main factors which reduce the loss of water from the skin – the outer horny layer or the stratum corneum and the invisible hydro-lipid film that covers the skin surface.

The flat overlapping dead cells of the stratum corneum make a somewhat water-proof cover, forming a natural barrier against excessive water loss. This layer contains chemical substances, which are the natural moisturising factors, which help to retain water in the skin. The other factor which prevents water loss is sebum. This forms a hydro-lipid film which holds onto the water. The degree of protection offered by sebum, however, varies depending on your skin type; it is maximum if your skin type is oily.

In an atmosphere with low humidity, such as during cold windy weather or with central heating or air-conditioning, the water tends to be drawn out of the skin into the surrounding air at a rate much faster than it can be replaced. Excessive exposure to the sun, especially if the skin is not protected by an appropriate screen, also dries the skin. Soaps and detergents reduce the ability of the skin to retain water, because they damage the natural moisturising factors and also remove the oil from the hydro-lipid film. Using cosmetic cleansers, unsuitable for your skin type can also dehydrate your skin; for instance, a product formulated to clean and remove excess oil from an oily skin can play havoc with dry skin because it would further remove the oil and reduce its ability to hold water.

When insufficient water is present in the skin, it becomes rough, dry, flaky and fragile — this type of skin looks rather unattractive. If allowed to further lose moisture, the skin cracks up and becomes painful — such skin is in urgent need of artificial moisturisers.

Your skin and the sun

Energy from the sun reaches the earth as rays of various wavelengths, some short and some long. Wavelengths shorter than visible light are known as ultraviolet rays; two different types of these penetrate the earth's atmosphere — the UVA and the UVB.

Although ultraviolet rays are invisible, they have several effects on the skin. UVB increases pigmentation through increased production of melanin. The other response of the skin, to exposure to ultraviolet rays, is thickening. Both these changes provide a natural barrier, protecting the skin from the more serious side-effects of the sun.

Over the years, the skin also shows many other changes: wrinkles, excessive dryness and irregularities in the skin colour and texture. The skin becomes thick and the bundles of collagen (which give the skin elasticity) become less evenly distributed. So the skin loses its suppleness and becomes wrinkled. There are also other effects of sunlight. Some people develop irregularities of the skin of the hands and face known as keratoses — these should never be ignored as they can become cancerous.

Individuals of the darker races have a natural protection from the deleterious effects of the sun, because of the presence of large amounts of melanin in their skin. But fair-skinned people have only a limited natural protection from sun rays, and therefore, need other means to guard themselves. There are several ways of doing this:

- Wearing apparel could be modified.
- You could use sun-shades and umbrellas.
- Use protective sunscreens.

Sunscreens

Protective creams or sunscreens work in two ways — they either reflect off the ultraviolet rays or they absorb the rays before they can do any damage (Table 1). *Calamine lotion* and thick creams, such as *zinc oxide* cream, work in the first way; but for them to work, they need to be applied in a thick layer and so are generally not cosmetically acceptable. The absorbent type of sunscreens selectively absorb UVB, and some UVA. This category includes benzophenones and cinnamates because these are not visible, they are cosmetically acceptable and so are very popular. Para aminobenzoic acid is no longer used, because it causes allergic reactions.

Table 1. Sunscreens and their properties.

Physical sunscreens	Chemical sunscreens
Zinc oxide (calamine) Titanium dioxide	Benzophenones Cinnamates
Broad spectrum (reflect all light)	Not so broad spectrum i.e., selective
Visible, so cosmetically not acceptable	Invisible, so cosmetically acceptable
No allergic reaction	Allergic reactions can occur

Are sunscreens perfectly safe? Most of the time yes! Sunscreens, like calamine lotion, are very safe, except that they cause slight dryness of the skin. This variety of sunscreens, however, is not used frequently, as they are cosmetically not acceptable.

POINTS TO REMEMBER WHEN USING A SUNSCREEN

When and how to use?

Sunscreens need to be used several times a day, because they get washed away even by sweat. We tell our patients to apply them at 8 AM, 12 noon and 4 PM. If you are likely to be under fluorescent lights (tubelights/arc lights) in the evening or at night, then you may need another application at night. Remember the whole face and any other part of the body exposed to sunlight needs to be protected.

SPF of sunscreen

This is a frequently used term when a sunscreen is purchased. It means the *Sun Protecting Factor* of the sunscreen. SPF is a crude way of defining the number of times the sun exposure can be increased following application of the sunscreen. So SPF 15 means you can increase the sun exposure 15 times before your skin becomes red on exposure to sunlight.

CLEANSING YOUR SKIN

When to clean your face?

Skin must be cleansed frequently enough or infrequently enough, depending on its needs. It really does not matter when you clean it: most people do this as the first thing in the morning and the last thing at night, simply because these times are convenient. Scientifically, going to bed in your make-up really will do your skin no harm, but it certainly won't do your bed linen any good. And since it is much easier to remove make-up from the face than from the linen, it would seem wiser to cleanse your face before going to bed. In the morning, cleansing the skin is very refreshing. Also, if you have to apply make-up, you would get a better 'finish' on the just cleansed skin.

How often must you clean your face?

Most people do this 2-3 times a day; this is adequate for normal skins. But, if your skin is oily or if you are exposed to a lot of grime and dirt during the course of the day, a more frequent cleaning is very essential — even 4-5 times a day may be necessary, using either a soap or some kind of cleansing agent.

If, on the other hand, your skin is dry, too frequent cleaning may harm it, especially if you use very hot water. With this skin type, it is best to avoid too frequent washing and you may even have to use a suitable oil-based cosmetic cleanser instead of soap, which has a drying effect.

How you clean your face is equally important. If at the end of the day cleansing involves removing make-up as well as grime and dirt that has accumulated during the day, then it should definitely be a thorough job. Provided you clean your face well at night, the morning session need not be too elaborate.

What should you use for cleansing?

Ordinary soap is often dismissed as useless and harmful by many people. This is absolutely untrue. The purpose of any cleansing operation (a term favoured by some skin-care people for a process most of us know as 'washing') is to remove dirt and grease. Ordinary soaps do this effectively (and sometimes even too thoroughly!). Soaps contain fats which work very effectively as cleansers of grease and grime. Soaps will also remove some cosmetics, but most of the heavily pigmented cosmetics and the water-proof eye make-up products are not easily removed with soaps — for these, a cosmetic cleanser is usually required.

You must always rinse the skin thoroughly with water after using soaps. Soap, if allowed to remain on the skin, attracts dirt; it can also cause irritation of the skin. In areas where the water is hard, soap residue if left on the skin can combine with the calcium and magnesium salts in the hard water to form a scum, and this is really very difficult to remove.

One unfortunate effect of soaps is that they remove some natural oils from the skin, making it dry. A related action is that, being alkaline, soaps neutralise the natural acidic film on the skin. Though these effects are temporary, they can cause problems in people with dry skin, during cold weather and in conditions of low humidity. The dryness, however, is easily countered by using a moisturising cream after washing with soap.

If your skin is dry, use soap and water for one cleanisng and at other times use a suitable cosmetic cleanser. However, in hot weather even a dry skin may tolerate several washings with soap and water. If you have a normal skin, then 2 to 3 washes with soap will not do your skin any harm, while an oily skin will benefit from an even more frequent cleansing with soap and water.

Which soap to choose?

In an attempt to corner profitable sections of the soap-buying market, manufacturers produce a variety of special soaps and advertise them making tall claims. Each one of us has wondered, at some time or the other, about which soap to buy. Here is a checklist to help you, when you next go soap-hunting.

Medicated soaps: These are often favoured by people who have spots. The medication usually added is an antiseptic (natural or synthetic). Actually, ordinary soap does a fairly good job of removing the bacteria from the surface of the skin. Medicated soaps do not further enhance the effect because they are in contact with the skin for a very, very short period. As a matter of fact, these soaps can, at times, cause allergic reactions (to the medication added) and are best avoided, unless your doctor specifically advises you to use them.

pH soaps: Soaps and detergents generally have an alkaline pH. If, because of its formulation, the pH of a soap falls near enough to neutral so as not to disturb the pH of the skin, then these soaps are called 'pH-controlled' soaps. The exact pH is sometimes stated on the label. Since the skin has a tremendous reserve, the pH altered by ordinary soaps is normally rapidly restored after thorough rinsing. So these pH-controlled soaps are only marginally superior to ordinary soaps.

Moisturising soaps: These do not have any advantage over other soaps because the rinsing, after the washing, removes the moisturising ingredients.

Superfatted soaps: These contain fatty materials (which are not saponified) to prevent excessive stripping of surface oils. They also deposit an emollient film to replace some of the natural oils removed in the cleansing process — these soaps can be used on dry skins.

Transparent soaps: These soaps are more difficult to prepare and so are expensive; they are not more effective or safer than ordinary soaps.

Liquid soaps: These are nothing but a dent in your pocket, because they offer no advantage over other soaps except being aesthetically appealing and less messy to use.

Perfumed soaps: These contain natural or artificial perfumes. They make you smell good. Sometimes, however, the perfumes may cause allergic reactions — so these soaps have their disadvantages too!

What are cleansing creams?

There are several alternatives to soap and water cleansing — creams, milks, lotions, foams, oils, gels and liquids. All these are rather closely related — much more than you can imagine. All are basically a mixture of oil, wax and water but manufacturers modify the formula to suit different skin types — those for dry skins remove less oil from the skin, and may even add some, whilst cleansers for oily skins are designed to remove more oil and add none to the skin.

It is also possible to clean your face equally efficiently with baby oil, liquid paraffin or vegetable oils. All of these remove make-up and dirt. But they are not pleasant-smelling. A cotton-pad dipped in fresh milk is a cheap but equally effective cleanser. If you do use any of these, and especially if you have an oily skin, it is necessary to wash the residue off with soap and water and to dab your face well with an astringent.

The right way to use a cleanser

Gently is the right way. Do not stretch, drag or pull your skin. It is important to remember that it is the cleanser which removes the make-up and not you; you only remove the cleanser, so do not be too vigorous in your attempts to either rub it in or to remove it.

With the cleanser in your hand, let your fingers glide over your skin, or use light patting movements with the pads of your fingers. Upward and outward movements have frequently been suggested as the right way to apply all kinds of creams to the face — this is thought to prevent or delay the eventual loss of muscle tone and the resultant sagging of the skin. Leave the cleanser on for a minute or two so as to loosen the dirt and make-up. Then gently remove it either with cotton wool or with tissue paper, again using upward and outward movements. Wipe over the face again with a damp cotton wool ball, and if it does not come away clean, repeat the cleansing process. Finally rinse with water.

Mechanical cleansing of your skin

A recent concept in skin cleansing is *epidermabrasion* — this is, literally, mechanically rubbing off the dead cells from the skin surface. Various substances are available — among the most familiar ones are a variety of granules (sand, sawdust, silica and pumice) and slowly soluble abrasive materials (like sodium tetraborate decahydrate). These granules can also be incorporated into soaps and creams and form the basis of some of the peeling face-masks available in the market. Other materials for epidermabrasion are sand-paper, hemp cloth, cellulose of the luffa plant, sea-sponges and man-made sponges of cellulose and polyurethane. Woven webs can also be used for epidermabrasion, the best known being the ubiquitous wash cloth, which provides a very delicate level of epidermabrasion. The most recent development in epidermabrasion technology is the use of non-woven polyester webs. Most skins tolerate this treatment well, though it should definitely be avoided on the very dry skins.

MOISTURISERS

How do moisturisers work?

Moisturisers are cosmetic products which to some extent provide a practical answer to problems of water loss from the skin. Though water is the missing ingredient, in dry skins, application of water alone is not the solution as this has only a temporary effect because it evaporates too fast! Though oil is equally essential (it serves to hold water on to the skin surface), it alone also can't moisturise the skin.

Moisturisers, therefore, combine both water and oil. This not only replaces some of the water lost from the skin, but more importantly prevents its loss to the surroundings. There are several moisturising products available in the market. They all fall, basically, into 2 main types: oil-in-water emulsions and water-in-oil emulsions.

The oil-in-water moisturisers sometimes also contain substances called *humectants* which attract water from the surroundings, but this may have its own disadvantage because humectants may sometimes absorb too much water from the skin itself, thereby increasing its dryness. A commonly used humectant is glycerine. Newer ingredients have been added to increase the efficacy of this group of moisturisers. Urea (which is an excellent fertilizer for soil) improves the efficiency of glycerine as a moisturiser.

A good household moisturiser can be prepared by dissolving 2 level teaspoons full of urea (can be procured from a garden shop) in 10 teaspoons of tap water and adding 10 teaspoons of glycerine.

The second category of moisturisers comprises the newer water-in-oil emulsions. They are marketed generally as creams or lotions. Being oil-based products, these trap moisture in the skin by forming an occlusive film on the skin surface; this forms a barrier retarding water loss. Many of these products are also called anti-dehydrating creams.

How to choose your moisturiser?

Choosing the moisturiser to best suit your skin type is very important. The proportion of oil varies according to the type of skin for which the product is formulated. The label on the product generally states this – so do read the instructions carefully!

Generally speaking, products meant for well-balanced normal skins are water-based, containing a little oil. Those designed for dry skins make up for the lack of oil in the skin, by adding oil to the skin. Humectants like glycerine and lactic acid, are also added to retain moisture. 'Sensitive' skins also need moisturisers having a high oil content.

Moisturisers are, generally, not to be used on oily skins, because they can cause spots. But today safe synthetic chemicals are available – these oil-free moisturisers do not contain any mineral oils, vegetable oils or animal fat, but contain either modified oils or other synthetic ingredients. So now you can enjoy the luxury of using such products, even if you have an oily skin. Use them on patches of dryness caused by excessive use of anti-pimple remedies. Don't use them too often or too liberally.

Now, newer light, non-greasy creams and lotions are also available – these are as effective as the heavy, thick and greasy creams and are competitively priced. They are the best type to be worn under make-up, as they give a superb finish to the make-up.

Is it worth using a moisturiser regularly?

Yes, regular use of a suitable moisturiser does benefit your skin. By guarding against the excessive loss of water, these agents protect the skin against the drying influences of the environment – the effects of sun, cold and heat. A moisturiser is particularly helpful for naturally dry skins, but whatever be your skin type, a moisturiser does compensate for the deficiencies in the natural oil-film and keeps the skin lubricated making it soft, smooth and looking more youthful.

Further, moisturisers give a smooth 'finish' to make-up. Putting on a light moisturising cream will make applying of make-up much easier and reduce the risk of 'dragging the skin'.

Most dermatologists agree that moisturisers effectively combat skin dryness and make the skin soft and supple. But the role of special ingredients, like vitamins, proteins, collagen and hormones, in many of the expensive creams is quite doubtful. In fact, it is only the simple lubricating action of the ingredients in the creams that do any good. So using exotic oils (such as deer oil) instead of ordinary oils, will not make the moisturiser any more effective, though it will add enormously to the cost. However, certain natural and synthetic substances, humectants like urea, lactic acid, and phospholipids, might improve the efficacy of moisturisers as they increase the hydration of the skin.

FEED YOUR SKIN

Massages

Done by experienced hands, a massage can help ease tension, soothe tight muscles and relieve pain. Remember, a massage should not be done on an inflammed skin and it should not be done without the use of oils or a light dusting of talc or baby powder to make the skin more malleable.

How often? You can give yourself a facial massage at least once a month. It is important that you relax and enjoy the total experience — the calmer you feel, the better will be the result. The massage should last about 10 minutes, anything longer will be too tiring.

What to use ? Always use a cream or oil suited to your skin type. An oil-free cream or baby powder is best for those with a greasy skin. A few drops of warm almond oil is a treat for dry skin.

Steps of the massage:

1. Tie your hair back, away from the face.
2. Apply the cream over the face and neck. Use powder for oily skins.
3. With your hands facing inward, start at the base of the neck and run your fingers lightly up, onto and over the face. Let the fingers of one hand follow those of the other, to the centre of the face (Fig. 3 A).
4. Using your index and middle fingers only, tap lightly all over the face.
5. With the thumb and index finger, gently knead the chin around the mouth and the fleshy part of the cheeks. Don't pull or pinch at the skin, but keep the movements firm, steady and even (Fig. 3 B).
6. Smooth and soothe the forehead by ironing over the fine lines. Hold the skin firm between the index and the middle fingers of one hand, and using the index finger of the other hand, massage the skin with inward and outward movements. Do this over the whole forehead (Fig. 3 C).
7. Using the same 2 fingers, massage the cheeks in circular movements (Fig. 3 D).
8. Now for the eyes: With the middle finger of each hand, gently smooth over the brow bone to the outside of the eye, then bring the fingers below the eyes and back to the centre. With the little finger, press around the outside of the eye especially where fine lines are present, and release immediately.
9. Repeat all the above steps thrice.
10. Finally close your eyes, and relax for a few minutes.
11. Remove the whole cream.

How does facial massage help?

Facial massage is a popular method, which has been used from time immemorial to improve the quality of facial skin. It has often been touted by the beauticians as a panacea for all ills of the face (a total exaggeration!). The cream massage increases the blood supply of the facial skin. This is thought to keep the skin supple and prevent premature aging of the skin. However, the greatest benefit of the massage is that it relaxes you and this effect is enhanced by adding aromatic oils.

Following the massage, the face may or may not be steamed. This is done using a hot towel or a steaming gadget and though the beautician may tell you that it opens the pores of the skin, steaming actually enhances the relaxation of the face and gives a feeling of warmth.

The present vogue of applying face packs has been attributed to a combination of the psychologic and cleansing effects of the face pack. The warmth and tightening resulting from the application produces a sensation of rejuvenation of the facial skin, whilst the colloidal and adsorptive clays and earths present in some of the packs adsorb skin debris, grease and dirt.

Problems after facial massage: Facial beauty treatments are soothing and relaxing procedures, but can definitely result in some problems:

- An eruption quite like acne can occur 4-6 weeks after a facial massage. In this, large pimples develop on the cheek and these heal after a long time leaving behind dark scars.
- Sometimes, exotic ingredients of the creams can cause allergic reactions.

Skin toners

This category of skin-care products includes cosmetics like skin fresheners, toners and astringents. They basically contain alcohol and water. Glycerine, witch hazel, menthol, camphor, boric acid, rose water and alum are often added. The basic difference in the formula is in the amount of alcohol these products contain. As alcohol has a very drying effect, there is little or none of it in the products intended for dry skin while the products for use on oily skin have a high alcohol content.

These products are used after cleaning the skin (with soap or any other cleanser), though they can be used as interim cleansers as well, as they can remove grime and oils. They freshen and tone up the skin and prepare it for application of make-up. They also restore the acid/alkali balance of the skin, because they are pH-balanced.

Despite claims to the contrary, fresheners, toners and astringents do not close pores. As a matter of fact, no cosmetic product can alter the actual size of the pores. What really happens after using these products is a mild irritation of the skin. This results in swelling of the skin and so the pores appear less prominent.

How do face masks help the skin?

Basically all face masks have some sort of a cleansing action. Various ingredients are used in the masks, depending on the skin type and to some extent on the availability of materials. Clays form an important

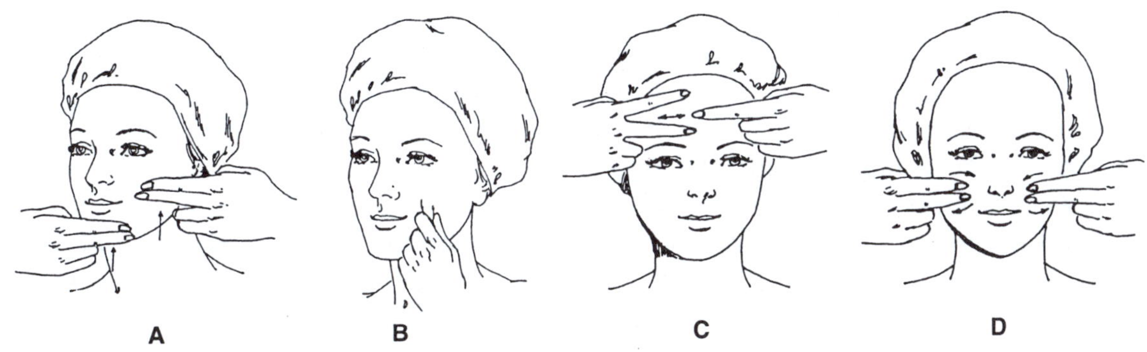

Fig. 3. Steps of an invigorating massage.

constituent of many face masks as they are excellent adsorbing agents. Gums and polymers are added to lend sticking properties to the clays. They help to remove dirt, sebum, and dead skin so that the skin looks clean, soft and youthful.

Fuller's earth is a special kind of clay often used in face packs. It contains aluminium silicate. As it dries on the skin, it adsorbs the superficial dead cells and blots up any excessive oil on the skin. It is therefore excellent for an oily skin but should not be used on a dry skin.

Kaolin is also a fine clay which has long been used for tummy upsets because it adsorbs toxins from the system. When used on the skin it removes grime, oils and dead cells. Kaolin is again ideally suited for oily skins and best avoided on dry skins.

Another ingredient of some of the masks is the peeling or the exfoliating agent — these remove the top layer of dead cells from the skin, leaving behind fresh youthful skin. They are usually well tolerated and brighten up a dull complexion. Oatmeal and bran are the commonly used peelers.

Oatmeal is obtained from oats. It is rich in vitamin B and vitamin E. For the last named content, it has been attributed with anti-aging qualities. However, it is quite unlikely that the contact for a short time, as during the application of the face pack, would benefit the skin. The rather youthful appearance of the skin after use of oatmeal containing masks is due to the removal of the superficial dead skin and the appearance of the younger skin on the surface. This effect is similar to the effect of epidermabrasion, a technique which we have already discussed.

Also added to many masks are natural ingredients — cucumbers, curds, lemon juice and Brewer's yeast. There are claims of several advantages of these additives; the one effect that has been scientifically established is the restoration of the acid/alkali balance of the skin by these agents as all of them have an acidic pH.

Use the mask to suit your skin

Identify your skin type before you apply the mask. It is best to try out a few of the masks suited to your skin type and discover for yourself, which of them is the most beneficial to you.

1. *For oily skin:* Mix 2 teaspoons of Fuller's earth with 2 teaspoons of chilled rose-water to make a thick paste. Apply on your face with a brush, avoiding the delicate areas around the eyes. Leave it on for about 20 minutes or till completely dry. Rinse with warm water. The result is a clear pinkish youthful skin – all the excess grease and dead cells have been cleared away. The treatment should be used for oily skins once a week but if your skin is really very oily then you can apply it even twice a week.
2. *For sallow looking oily complexions with blemishes:* Mix 3 teaspoons of kaolin with half a teaspoon each of rose-water, glycerine and tincture of benzoin; both kaolin and tincture of benzoin can easily be procured from the chemist. Apply the mask with a brush, leave it on for 30 minutes and wash it off with warm water. Your skin will appear soft and smooth with a glowing colour.
3. *Tonic for oily skin:* Whisk one egg white until it thickens, then whisk in 1 teaspoon of honey. Finally add 1 teaspoon of lemon juice. Apply to your face and neck avoiding the delicate eye and lip areas. Leave it on for 10 minutes and wash with warm water.
4. *Facial scrub for oily skin:* This is an invigorating way of cleansing the face, as the coarse texture of the scrub helps to get rid of the dirt and the superficial dead skin. It should not be used more than once a week and never on a dry skin. Mix 1 teaspoon of fine bran with a quarter teaspoon of dried yeast and 1 teaspoon of lemon juice along with a tablespoon of water. Gently massage the thick paste so formed into the skin, particularly on and around the nose and the chin area, using a soft brush; avoid applying around the eyes. Wash off after 1-2 minutes, using warm water.
5. *A moisturising pack for normal skin:* Mash or liquidise half an avocado pear with 1 teaspoon of sunflower oil. Apply the mixture to the face and neck avoiding the eye and lip area. Leave it on for 10 minutes and wash off with warm water.
6. *Toner for normal skin*: This is a refreshing toner for normal skins. Chop up a small size fresh cucumber and liquidise it with half a cup of yoghurt. Apply the mixture for 5-10 minutes, and wash it off. The remainder can be stored in the fridge for future use.
7. *Anti-aging mask for blotchy wrinkled skin:* This should be applied every other day. Mix 2 tablespoons of oatmeal with half a cup of milk and cook gently till it becomes soft. Stir in 2 teaspoons of olive oil and beat together. Allow to cool, then spread it over the face and neck. Leave it on, for about 25 minutes and then rinse away with lukewarm water.
8. *Rich pack for dry skin*: Whisk 1 egg white till it thickens, add 1 teaspoon of honey and 1 teaspoon of sunflower oil. Apply on the face for 20 minutes and wash off with warm water.

●●●

2. Make-up and the Art of Dressing up

Dressing up is not just the art of applying make-up – it is much more than that. It is truly a blend of art and science, requiring a spirit of adventure, the courage to experiment, an eye for colour harmony, some amount of perseverance, and the desire to look good. But since all these are present in you, just read on – follow the steps and you are sure to emerge a winner.

First of all, you must select your cosmetics – the colour and form of the make-up are both very important. Then you must prepare yourself for applying the make-up. Only then should you venture to apply make-up.

CHOOSING YOUR MAKE-UP WITH CARE

How to select the product?

Several points need to be considered here – your skin type and colour, your personality, the occasion, and last but not the least, the cost – all of these would influence the selection of your cosmetic products.

Your skin is the most important factor which should influence the selection of your cosmetics – the two aspects which need to be considered are: the skin type and the skin colour. Select cosmetics which suit your skin type; for instance, never purchase a cosmetic for oily skin if your skin type is dry because that would certainly be inviting trouble. Similarly, do not use cosmetics designed for dry skin if your skin type is oily.

The second aspect of choosing make-up is the harmony of colours. Colour harmony brings everything together, giving a well coordinated and agreeable effect. Any make-up you use should enhance your natural colouration, and not suppress it. The colour of your make-up should blend with the colour of your skin, your eyes and your hair.

There are two basic colour harmonies in make-up:

1. The bluish harmony or cold tones.
2. The gold harmony or warm tones.

Study the tones of your face thoroughly. Your face may have several colour tones – identify them and utilise the best colour harmony. Most of us in India have the gold harmony – yellow, beige, orange and brown tones with, perhaps, a tinge of green. People with the bluish harmony have blue, mauve, pink, reddish-blue and grey tones in their skin. Use only colours which complement your natural skin colour.

Another thing to remember is that not everyone can carry off heavy make-up. It is definitely better to look simply made-up, rather than grotesquely plastered. Also, your dress must suit your make-up and be just right for the occasion.

Why are some cosmetics so much expensive?

Although cosmetics are formulated from the same basic ingredients, the manufacturer does sometimes make a few additions and alterations — oils, for example, may be obtained from very inexpensive sources or may have terrifically esoteric origins. This single factor can rocket the price of the cosmetic, although, there is no proof to suggest that the expensive oils are in any way superior in performance to the cheaper ones.

Perfumes can also dramatically affect the cost of the product. Expensive perfumes will inflate the price of a cosmetic, without really improving its performance in any way. As a matter of fact, perfumes are a frequent cause of allergic reactions.

The addition of some other exotic substances can also hike up the price. Packaging and advertising greatly influence the cost of the product. The amount of scientific and technical expertise that has gone behind the product can greatly escalate the price. Finally, the brand name greatly influences the amount of money you are going to pay for the product.

FOUNDATIONS AND BLUSHERS

What are foundations?

Facial make-up or foundations are pigmented products intended for application on the face and the neck. They colour the skin evenly and hide facial imperfections such as scars, depressions and dark and light coloured areas.

Foundations come in several forms like emulsions, creams, liquids, gels, cakes and powders — these different forms contain the same basic ingredients, but differ in texture and finish, because the components are present in different proportions.

The basic formulation of the foundation is based on colouring agents (usually derived from iron oxide or titanium oxide), a wax (which gives an even flow and smooth finish), some form of cellulose (to make the foundation thick and adherent), an emulsifier, preservatives, and usually a perfume.

Effects created by different foundations. Which foundation should you select?

Several forms of foundations are available. You must choose your foundation correctly and for this you need to know the effect of each of the forms.

Emulsions: These are packaged in tubes and are formulated for a variety of skin types — for dry skins, oily skins and normal skins. They give less sheen than cream or liquid foundations, but cover blemishes very well.

Creams: These are packaged in jars. As they contain a high proportion of oils, they are particularly suitable for dry skins. These also provide a heavy cover, but give a glossy finish.

Liquids: These are packaged in bottles and can be formulated for all skin types — so look at the label before you purchase! Along with the cake variety, they are the commonest type of foundation used. They give a light sheen cover but are too light to cover any blemishes and scars.

Gels: These are packaged in squeeze tubes. They give a light, natural look and are the variety you should use if you have a blemish free normal skin.

Cakes or sticks: These are the solid forms of foundation. Since they have a drying effect, use them on an oily skin. They give a dense matt cover and are good for covering blemishes and scars. Solid forms are popular for photographic and stage work but are too heavy for everyday use.

Powders: The original full coverage face-powders have now given way to transparent powders; these transparent powders control shine and provide oil blotting. They are used after foundations to give a matt finish. Cake or compact powders are more heavily formulated; as they contain certain amount of foundation, these are not the best choice for the initial powdering over foundation because they may rub the foundation off and also cause an unattractive colour build-up. They are best used for touching up during the day, when they help to reinforce coverage.

Are foundations bad for your complexion?

The answer is a definite no. As a matter of fact, they are really good for the skin: they act as a barrier for the skin protecting it against dirt, wind and environmental pollutants; they also act as sun-screens guarding the skin against the ill-effects of the sun. Since foundations also contain moisturising agents, they balance the moisture levels of the skin. At the same time, they also act as an all-day blotting agent controlling the facial oiliness. Some foundations may even contain medication to dry up pimples.

Psychologically, the effects of foundation are dramatic too! They help in improving your looks: they even out tones, improve skin colour and texture, and disguise blemishes — all true morale boosters, working wonders for your confidence.

The idea that foundation may be harmful for the skin is based on the wrong notion that it blocks the skin pores (where sweat glands and sebaceous glands open); as a result it is thought that the skin cannot breathe and perspire. This concept is absolutely ridiculous, because make-up is not airtight, so it definitely cannot occlude the skin pores and so does not affect the functioning of the skin glands at all.

However, if you use a foundation which does not suit your skin type, you might develop problems: for instance, if you have an oily skin and you use a foundation formulated for dry skin (containing more oil), you could develop pimples. This can easily be remedied by changing over to a suitable preparation.

Rarely, however, you may develop an allergy to the foundation, in which case you should either stop using foundation or change over to somewhat safer *hypo-allergic* products.

Choosing your foundation

There are two aspects of foundations which require selection – the form and the colour. The first thing you have to decide on, is the form of the foundation. Some forms are more suited to certain skin types than others. A dry skin is best served by an oil-based foundation (cream type) as this gives additional moisture. An oily skin requires a less oily foundation – even an oil-free, water-based one (cake or stick form). For normal skin it is easy to choose. Emulsions and liquid foundations can be formulated to suit all skin types. So you must stick to the recommendations on the label.

Skin type apart, age and the basic condition of your skin would also influence the choice of your foundation. The better the condition of the skin, the thinner should the foundation be; so light sheer liquids are good on young or fine skins. A light liquid may also be the best choice for an older skin, though two coats may be required to give full coverage; a heavier product on such a skin may emphasise the lines and the skin creases. If your skin is in a poor condition (has an uneven colour or tone or is blemished) then a heavier foundation (cream or stick) will give a better appearance. If you have a fine skin and you want a natural appearance, then use the gel foundations.

If you are already using a foundation but are not sure to which category it belongs, you can find this out by putting a drop of the foundation into a dish of water. If the foundation disperses easily and can be stirred into the water to form a cloudy liquid, it is predominantly water-based and can be used if you have an oily skin; if, however, it remains in a blob and on stirring breaks up into smaller blobs, it is oil based and should be used on dry skins and not on oily skins.

The next thing is to choose the colour. From a wide variety of colours now available, it should not be too difficult to choose a shade that matches the natural colouring of your face. A harmonised make-up base must match the natural skin tone of the person as much as possible – for the gold harmony of skin colour use beige, brownish-gold or ochre and for the bluish harmony use pinkish-beige, peach or pinkish ochre.

If there are more than one colour tones in your face then match the foundation to the middle tone. This colour matching is best done in day-light and not in artificial light. While choosing colour of the foundation, it would be ideal to test it on your face, failing which, the next best area to match is the inside of your wrist.

Mixing two foundation colours – one which matches your skin and the other which complements your natural colouring could have a dramatic effect. The complementary colours should be chosen with equal care: unattractive skin tones like red can be balanced by a beige tone, while a slightly pink foundation will warm a sallow complexion.

Use of a blusher

After facial make-up, the next thing that comes on the face is the blusher. This is a highlighting colour, that is applied on the high edge of the cheek bones and is blended to create a natural-looking blush on the cheeks. The predominant form today is the powder blusher — this is the successor to the original rouge. Cream blushers are somewhat newer than powder blushers. Blushers also come in two colour harmonies: the gold harmony with coral, orange and reddish brown tones and the bluish harmony with rose-beige colours. Remember that here too you must select both the right form and the right colour.

EYE-COSMETICS

How safe are eye-cosmetics?

The regulations governing the manufacture of eye cosmetics should, ideally, be very strict. Only those chemicals which will definitely not cause any damage to the eyes, should be used. The preservatives in eye-cosmetics must not only be safe, but also be strong enough to preserve the product.

Most instances of infection and injury to the eyes are a result of careless application and use of cosmetics rather than due to any of its ingredients. So it is important to follow simple rules of cleanliness and hygiene when using eye-cosmetics: wash your hands before touching your eyes; never borrow or lend any item of eye make-up; never use saliva or dirty water to moisten eye make-up.

Allergic reactions to eye make-up are, however, not uncommon; the solution to this problem is to stop using the eye-cosmetic which has caused the reaction. But, remember that reactions around the eyes are not always due to eye-cosmetics, but may be due to the nail varnish or the hair-dye you have used. A myth that really needs to be dispelled is that eye-cosmetics cause eyelashes to fall out. Like all body hair, your eyelashes grow, fall off and are replaced cyclically. It is just that while you are using eye-cosmetics you tend to become aware of this loss and you may wrongly blame the cosmetics.

Choosing eyeshadows for yourself

The eyeshadow you choose should flatter and enhance your eye colour and the shape of your eyes, as well as your whole appearance. The skin colour, the eye colour, and your lifestyle need to be considered when choosing and using eyeshadow. Although there are no hard and fast rules for choosing the colour of your eyeshadow it is best to find out by experimenting with colours. But always harmonise the colour of the eyeshadow with that of your skin and your eyes. Whatever the colour, it should be blended in well, so that there are no harsh lines. Aim always for a natural look.

Apart from colour, there is a choice of forms of the eyeshadows. You can choose from pressed powders, pencils, sticks, gels, crayons and creams. Pressed powders are still the most popular form of shadows, because they are easy to apply and control. These are available in pearly and matt textures. The effect is not long lasting, but if you apply them with a wet brush, you can get a deeper effect and increase the staying qualities of the colour.

The cream shadows are oil or wax based. They are best suited for dry crepey lids and should be avoided on greasy lids. Sticks are a firmer form of cream shadow and look quite like lipsticks. Pencils have, however, almost totally replaced sticks and crayons. They have a high colour and filling ability. Gels are suited for greasy skins. These give a long lasting, subtle and translucent effect. Liquid shadows also have a long lasting effect, but are difficult to apply because it is difficult to get an even flow of colour with them.

Lining the eyes

Eyeliners, including our own indigenous *kaajal* are the most extensively used form of eye make-up. Liners outline the eye and are particularly attractive in deeper toning colours (to match the eyeshadow).

The earlier cake type of liner has now been somewhat replaced by liquids and pencils. The liquid liners are sold in bottles either with a separate sable brush or in an automatic-unit with the brush built into the cap. The product may be either water-based (when it is susceptible to wetting with water) or alcohol-based (when it is water-proof). Our own *kaajal* has also undergone a considerable improvement—from cake to stick and now to a pencil, which is so easy to use.

Mascara

Mascara coats the lashes, making them thick, long, lustrous and more noticeable. You can choose from 3 different forms of mascara – water-based, water-proof and the mixed variety.

Water-based mascaras can be applied quickly because they dry rapidly. They can also be removed easily, so they are gentle to the lashes and the eyes. But there are several problems with their use: because the water evaporates quickly, the lashes tend to clump together; as the film is not water-proof, the mascara smudges easily when it comes in contact with water, tears, and perspiration; because of the high water content, these products are difficult to preserve and have a short shelf life.

Because of these disadvantages of water-based mascaras, the water-proof variety has become popular. Water-proof mascaras are generally long wearing, water-proof and smudge-proof; but they are difficult to remove and you may have to use a cosmetic cleaner to remove them. Because they take long to dry, they have a tendency to smear unless you are careful. Though they colour and appear to lengthen the lashes well, they do not thicken them much. They are, however, a good investment, because they are resistant to contamination and can be used even years after they have been manufactured.

The third variety of mascara is a combination of the earlier two types. These dry quickly, produce little or no smudging and are the latest in the field of mascaras.

The under-eye concealers

The under-eye concealers are intended to hide blemishes, imperfections and dark circles under the eyes. They are more opaque than regular make-up, but still need to be matched to the skin tone. They are so formulated that the subsequent application of make-up does not remove them.

AN ARRAY OF COSMETICS FOR LIPS

The colour of your lips brightens and enhances your appearance! It is the final touch to facial make-up. Lip cosmetics are now available in sticks, tubes, pencils, as liquids and in pots.

Why should a liplining pencil be used?

A liplining pencil has a harder consistency than a lipstick and is used to outline the lips so as to clearly define their shape. It is a great aid, if your lips are not perfectly shaped: you can make the lips appear thinner or fuller or you can draw an uplifted corner if your lips droop. The outlining of the lips, in addition, prevents bleeding of the lip product into the tiny lines that are present around the mouth, giving the lips a sharp, defined outline.

Your lipsticks

Lipsticks are the most commonly used lip make-up. They come in a variety of colours. The colour you use should harmonise not only with the rest of the make-up but with your attire and with the rest of you as well. Remember, pale skins would need soft colours while darker skins can carry off the more vibrant shades.

Most lipsticks consist of a fatty base to ensure that the product stays firm and solid. At the same time, efforts are made to make the product soft enough to cover the lips smoothly and with minimum of pressure. The colour in the lipsticks is provided by pigments or dyes. These should not fade off too quickly but should stay on the lips while you eat, drink, smoke and kiss. It is also equally important that no unsafe chemicals are used as the product is often swallowed.

Why does the colour of lipstick change on the lips?

When your lipstick changes colour or 'turns blue' on your lips, after a period of wear, it is an indication that it needs to be reapplied. This change occurs because the so-called true colour of the lipstick (the colour you see in the lipstick case or on the lips immediately after application) has worn out more quickly than those components of the lipstick which are responsible for the adherence and these chemicals generally have a slight bluish tone.

Habits like biting or picking the lips intensify the problem, since they help remove the true colour even more quickly. If your lips are not dry and clean, when you are applying the lipstick, the colour loss is more rapid. You would face this problem less frequently with brown or brick shades, since these pigments tend to keep their colour better than pink or mauve shades.

Lipsticks seem to come off rather easily nowadays as they are less heavy and less staining than they once were. This is because they contain more waxes and emollients to give them a sheer glossy finish — something which today's consumer wants.

SPECIAL COSMETICS

Hypoallergic cosmetics for sensitive skins

The term hypoallergic cosmetics means less likely to cause an allergic reaction. They are a good substitute when they have to be used on sensitive skins. They do not contain the chemicals which commonly cause allergies; for instance, they do not contain perfumes.

If your skin has a tendency to develop allergic reactions and if you are trying out a new brand of cosmetic for the first time, purchase only small quantities of the product. Further, test its suitability on your skin. This is easily done by trying a simple patch test on the skin. Apply a small amount of the cosmetic onto a piece of cloth and fix this onto your skin – it does not matter where you stick this test patch, as long as it is on a part which you can inspect afterwards; also the site should not be too noticeable if you develop an unsightly rash.

Leave the cloth on for 48 hours. If on removing the cloth, you find that you have developed a red itchy rash, you are probably allergic to the cosmetic and definitely should not use it. Once you find cosmetics which are suited to your skin, we would advise you to stick to them. Remember that if you have a sensitive skin, it is worthwhile not to be too adventurous.

Herbal cosmetics

Herbal cosmetics have become extremely popular in the last couple of decades. Several people are now manufacturing and marketing them on a large scale. Individuals are also making their own cosmetics at home, either with ingredients they have bought or with substances 'off the kitchen shelf'. There is definitely something rather attractive about being able to get back to nature and to use natural cosmetics. But a couple of points need to be remembered:

- Do not imagine that just because a cosmetic is herbal or natural, it cannot produce an allergic reaction. It can and it often does.
- Be on the lookout for confidence tricksters. Do not automatically believe that just because there are pretty flowers on the label, the product is very natural.
- Remember that herbal products do not contain preservatives. This means that they cannot be kept for long periods. They should, therefore, be prepared or bought only in small quantities and used very soon.

Fairness creams

Beauty has often been equated with fairness. Therefore, a lot of effort and research has been put into the discovery and production of fairness creams. The fairness creams available have 2 important ingredients: an agent which decreases the production of melanin pigment in the skin; the agent most commonly used is *hydroquinone*. The other agent is a sunscreen which prevents the darkening effect of sunlight on the skin colour.

However, a note of caution on the fairness creams: some fairness creams actually contain a derivative of hydroquinone instead of hydroquinone (monobenzyl ether of hydroquinone). This chemical is very dangerous because it permanently kills the melanocytes (the pigment producing cells of the skin) causing leucoderma.

PREPARATION OF THE FACE FOR MAKE-UP

For the best final result, you must meticulously prepare your face for the actual application of the make-up.

Identify the structure of your face

This is very important, so that you can understand the high points and the drawbacks of your face. Then you will be able to emphasise the excellent features of your face and camouflage your handicaps.

Faces are of 2 basic shapes: angular and round. Angular faces are well delineated, with a strong bone structure and musculature. Angular faces (Fig. 4 A–D) could be trapezoidal, rectangular, square or triangular. Round faces, on the other hand, have curved, continuous, gently sloping lines, without any bony projections. Round faces (Fig. 4 E and F) can be oval or the true round form.

The ideal shape of a face is oval. So with the clever use of make-up, you must attempt to make your face appear oval. This can be done by using foundations of different tones — the dark shades (brown or bister) and the pale shades (white or clear). Dark make-up tends to reduce, deepen, darken and conceal and is suitable for contouring prominent cheeks, large noses, chubby faces, and for the bags under the eyes. Pale make-up, on the other hand, enlarges, lengthens, brightens, fills out, and covers the dark circles under the eyes.

Getting ready

Before applying make-up, especially if you are dressing for a rather important occasion, you must prepare yourself in a very special way. Massage your face with a nourishing cream, follow it up with a suitable mask. See that there are no dark hair visible on the face — bleach them or pluck them, if necessary. You might need to remove unwanted hair from your arms, legs and underarms.

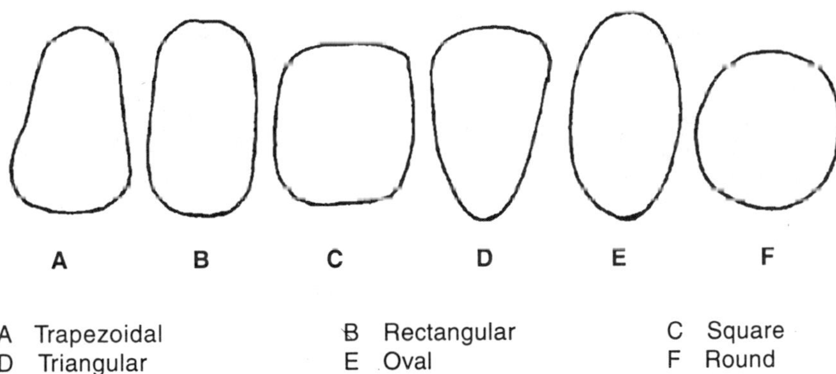

A Trapezoidal B Rectangular C Square
D Triangular E Oval F Round

Fig. 4. Identify the shape of your face.

Shaping your eyebrows

Eyebrows give the face its expression. So it is really worth spending some time deciding on the shape and contour of your eyebrows. But, if you think that you would require a drastic change in the shape of your brows, it would be best to seek professional help, at least for the first time.

The single-most important point to remember when shaping your eyebrows is the balance. Your facial shape would, to a large extent, determine the shape of your eyebrows. Here are some tips to help you decide on the shape of your brows:

For a trapezoidal face: Slightly thicken the eyebrows drawn gently towards the temple.

For a rectangular face: Keep the eyebrows as natural as possible.

For a square face: Give a slightly rounded curve.

For a triangular face: Brows should not be too thick. Curve the brows slightly upwards, to emphasise the triangular shape of the face.

For an oval face: Keep the brows parallel to the lid and drawn towards the temple.

For a round face: Brows should be slightly arched, in an oblique curve directed towards the temple.

Where to begin and where to end (Fig. 5): Take a pencil and hold it vertically alongside the outer corner of the nostril; the point where the pencil touches the eyebrow is the starting point. Then slant the pencil from the outer corner of the nostril to the outer corner of the eye, to show you where the arch should end. Then look straight ahead — the highest point for the eyebrows should be directly above the iris. Ideally, the distance between the two eyebrows should be equal to the width of one eye.

Getting the shape right: Before you start plucking, check your tweezers — buy those types which have slanted or squared off ends and a good grip. Begin by brushing the eyebrows upward with a clean mascara brush.

When shaping the brows, always pluck from beneath and never from above. Hold the skin taut with your first and second

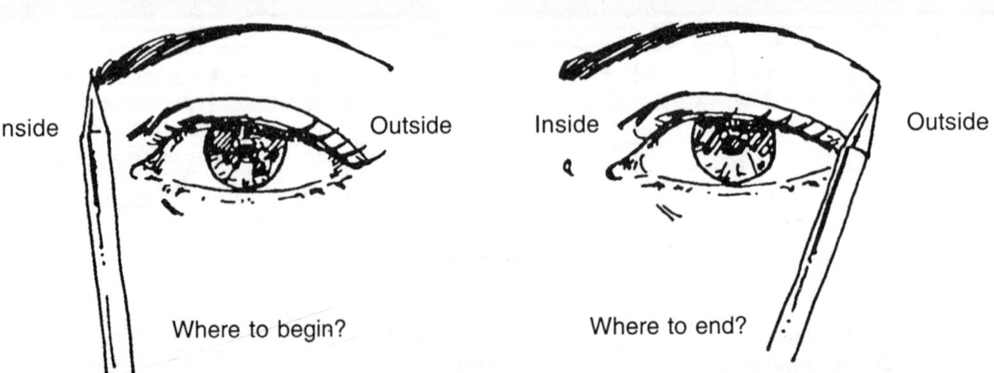

Fig. 5. Shaping your eyebrows.

fingers. Hold each hair as closely as possible to the roots and pluck in the direction of the hair growth. Plucking against the direction of the growth can cause the hair to break off at the skin surface and then it reappears very soon. Plucking in the wrong direction can also distort the follicle or the root – this results in the hair growing out at different angles.

First remove any stragglers in between the brows; then tidy the general outline. Absolutely avoid the use of scissors. Finally, brush the eyebrows again, wipe them with a mild toner and finish off with a moisturiser to soothe the skin. Avoid applying make-up immediately.

Cleansing of the face

For a glowing end-result, it is necessary to use the make-up on a really clean skin. The cleansing operation frees the skin of the stale make-up, dirt, dead cells and skin secretions.

What to use for cleansing? This depends on your skin type and also on whether you want to use readymade cleansers or you want to use home-made cleansers. From the market you can purchase a cleanser suited to your skin type; for instance, if you have a dry skin, you must choose an oil-based cleansing lotion. For those of you, who favour natural products, I have found fresh milk a very effective skin cleanser.

Pour a small quantity of cleansing agent onto a cotton ball. Cleanse the lips and then the area around the eyes; begin gently with the eyelashes and then clean the lids, starting on the upper lid near the nose, work outwards with a circular movement and come back towards the nose under the eye.

Using another cotton ball, dipped in the cleanser, clean the neck and the face in the steps as shown in Figure 6. At first, it all seems rather complex, but after a couple of times you will master the steps and then the whole process of cleansing will become automatic. It will then not take more than a couple of minutes. Finally, rinse thoroughly with warm water.

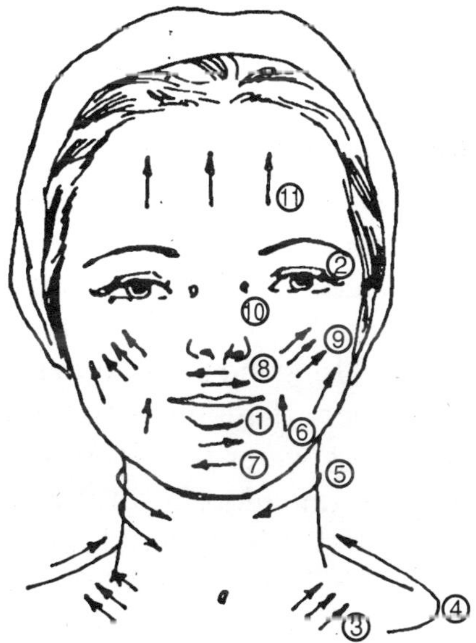

Fig. 6. Cleansing of the skin.

THE ACTUAL APPLICATION OF MAKE-UP

Make-up should be applied in the following sequence:

1. Foundation, preceded, if required, by under-eye concealers.
2. Corrections and improvements.
3. Blushers.
4. Powders.

5. Eye make-up.
6. Lip make-up.

Foundations

Foundations are designed to give a soft, even, natural glow to the face. The best coverage comes with the use of the right colour and product type and not from the amount of foundation you apply. Get your foundation base right – in form, in colour, and in application – and you have truly laid a foundation to a dazzling look – a smooth and perfectly toned canvas on which you can create a really beautiful picture.

Application technique

Put a little foundation on the hand (add a complementary tone, if necessary). Dot it over the face – on the nose, the cheeks, the chin and the temples and in between the brows. Using the tips of two fingers or a small, clean, dampened sponge (from which excess water has been removed), blend the foundation. Always work from the face outwards to avoid an accumulation of the foundation around the hairline – move from the cheeks to the ears, from the temples up and out to the hairline, from between the brows down over the nose, from the chin out towards the jaw, then onto the neck (Fig. 7).

Work quickly, carefully and lightly. Blend well around the hairline, on the neck, below the eyes and behind the ears. Also take the foundation over the eyelids. Finally blot the face with a clean dry tissue, pressing it lightly over the skin.

Use of under-eye concealers: Concealers are applied to cover dark circles around

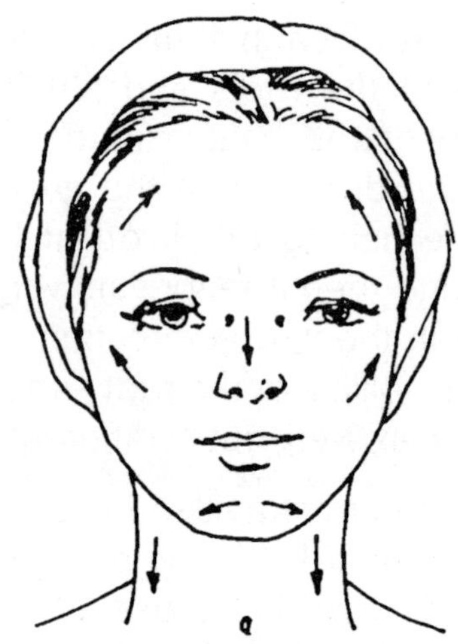

Fig. 7. Blending your foundation.

the eyes, thereby greatly enhancing the appearance of the face. They are matched to the skin tone and are applied before using the harmony foundation. When any product is applied around the eyes, special care must be taken so that the skin is not stretched. Instead of applying the cream from the inside corner of the eye to the outside, it should be dabbed on the skin and then gently blended with the finger tips moving from the outside corner to the inside corner. This procedure will not pull the skin. Position the concealer as shown in Fig. 8. After the product has dried, more can be applied to build up the desired opacity. To remove, use a cosmetic cleanser, instead of vigorously rubbing the skin with soap and water.

Corrections and improvements through the use of make-up

No woman is totally happy with her looks and most would like to make a few changes. With a bit of know-how and some initiative you can work wonders with your appearance; you can correct poor

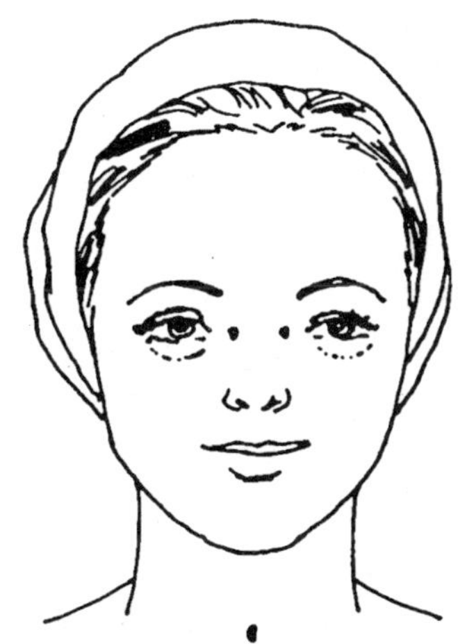

Fig. 8. Positioning of under-eye concealer to camouflage dark circles.

tones of the skin as well as improve your facial morphology.

Correction of poor skin tones is achieved by using a correcting make-up base: a mauve base can conceal pale and dull skin tones and brighten the skin. A green base masks red blotches and ruddiness. The under-eye concealer camouflages dark circles under the eye. These correcting bases have to be applied before applying foundation.

To improve facial features, use is made of the fact that pale shades lengthen, fill out, and brighten, while dark shades reduce, deepen, darken, and conceal. This form of correcting base is applied after the use of basic foundation. These correcting bases are available as liquids, creams and even as pencils.

1. *Correcting the facial morphology:* The ideal facial shape is oval and by the clever use of dark and pale tones, every facial type can be made to appear oval (Fig. 9).

A. The trapezoidal face can be made to look more oval by redefining the lower part with dark foundation and using light make-up at the temple (Fig. 9A).

B&C. The rectangular and square shapes are redefined at the four corners with dark foundation (Fig. 9B and C).

D. The triangular face needs dark foundation at the temples and to shorten the chin while the lower face needs enlargement using light make-up (Fig. 9D).

E. The oval face needs shortening at the forehead and chin with dark foundation (Fig. 9E).

F. The round face is made to appear oval by using dark make-up at the temples and around the lower face (Fig. 9F).

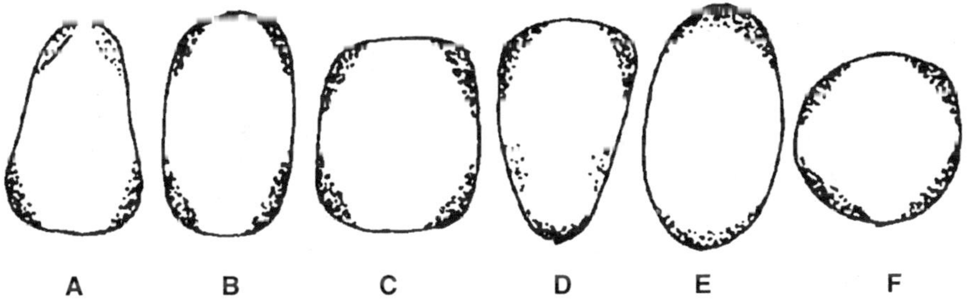

Fig. 9. Correcting facial morphology.

2. *Correcting the chin and the nose:* Here again, playing with colours, you can balance other features of your face (Fig.10).

A. A prominent chin can be corrected by applying dark foundation on the tip of the chin (Fig.10A).

B. A double chin can be corrected by putting a dark foundation on the double chin (Fig.10B).

C. A long nose appears short by applying dark make-up on the tip (Fig.10C).

D. For a broad nose apply dark foundation along each side of the nose (Fig.10D).

E. To emphasise a short nose apply pale make-up along the top of the nose along its whole length (Fig.10E).

F. For a narrow nose apply a bright foundation on each side (Fig.10F).

G. For a crooked nose, cover the crooked side with a dark foundation and the opposite side with a light foundation (Fig.10G).

Applying blusher

The next step is the use of the blusher or the rouge. These cosmetics do several things to your face. They add shape, and definition to your face, giving your complexion a wonderful, warm and youthful glow. Blushers are available as powders, creams and sticks. Powder blushers are brushed on the face after powdering the face, while the cream and the stick varieties are applied after the foundation, but before using the powder.

To apply: Use the colour on the blush area (Fig. 11). This is the part of the face between parallel lines, one extending outward from the corner of your eye and the second from the bottom of your nose. A touch of colour across the forehead and on the chin completes the look. The cream rouge is applied to the cheeks with the fingertips in small amounts and spread in the desired fashion. The powder blusher is applied with a brush.

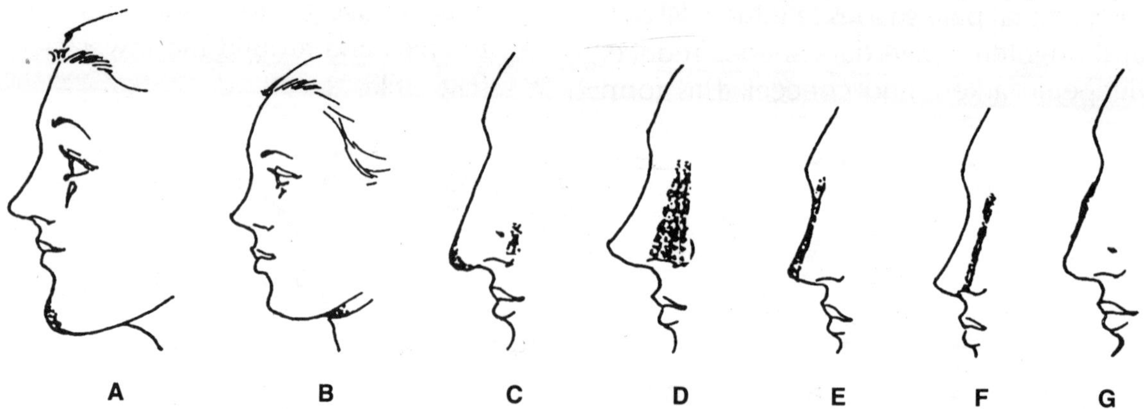

Fig. 10. Contouring the chin and the nose.

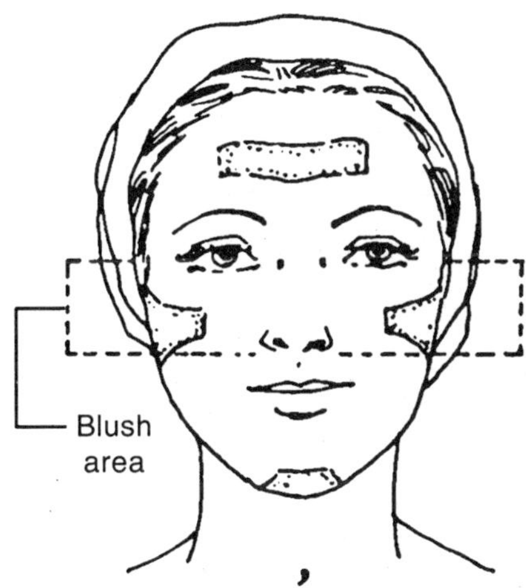

Fig. 11. Positioning of blusher on the face.

Use of powder — setting your make-up

Powder does two things to your make-up. Firstly, it sets your make-up perfectly, giving a smooth, even finish to the complexion. Secondly, it helps to prevent the appearance of shine on the areas most prone to oiliness — the central panel. Applied correctly, your make-up will stay fresh throughout the day.

Which powder to use?: Fine loose translucent powders are the best, as the pressed powders tend to cake and streak. Avoid the tinted ones as these colour the face rather brightly and grey with time on the face.

Technique: Make sure the foundation is well blended. Blot the face lightly with a tissue, especially over the forehead, nose and chin. Pick up the powder on the puff and press it firmly on the face, one area at a time. Don't try to smooth it on by massaging the puff over the face. Now using a soft, thick powder brush, whisk away the excess, with downward movement to stop the powder getting caught in the fine facial hair.

Eye make-up

Making the eyes come alive is a real art and like any good artist you will have to first learn the techniques of accurate brush work and careful colour-blending. Almond shaped eyes are considered to be ideal. So when making-up eyes, one tries with the help of light and dark eye make-up to make the necessary changes to give the eyes an almond-like appearance.

Eyeshadow

Eyeshadow comes in various forms: pressed powders, loose powders, creams, sticks and as liquids. Pressed powders are the easiest to apply.

Application: (Fig.12). The following steps are followed in the application of eyeshadow shades:

1. Using a fine, blunt-ended brush, gently apply the base colour to the entire lid from the inside to the outside corner and from the base of the lashes to the eyelid crease (Fig. 12A).

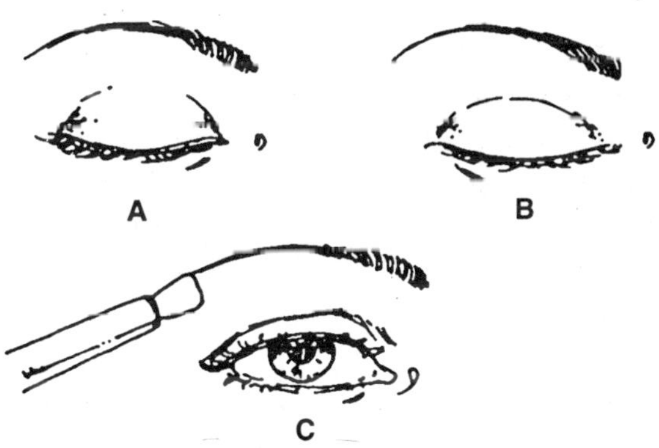

Fig. 12. Application of eyeshadow.

2. If the eyes need extra definition, a deeper shade is blended into the crease line. This gives depth to the eyes (Fig.12B).
3. The brow bone is highlighted with a light shade. This gives the eyes a wide, open look. The colour is applied to the most prominent area and blended up towards the brow and down to where the contour curves down, towards the eyelid creases (Fig.12C).

Before using them on the lids, always test the colours on the back of the hand to see the intensity. You can use even 3-4 colours, provided they are blended well. Remember, pale tones emphasise, while deep sooty shades define.

Use of liners – adding depth to your eyes

Depth and intensity, drama and expression come to the eyes through the clever use of definers: eyeliners, pencils and kohls. Available in rich, dark shaded colours, these emphasise the eyes, create new shapes and give the eyes a mysterious and exotic allure. Here again, practice will make you perfect.

Using the liquid liner: (Fig.13). Test on the back of your hand the amount of pressure you should apply. Unless you are a real artist, it is best to steady your elbow on a flat surface. Work from the inside of the eye to the outside corner and keep the line light and even. If you stop at the corner of the eyes, the effect will be round and wide-eyed; if you continue the line and sweep it up and out, you would get a more exotic look. Finally smudge the edges with a cotton bud to soften them.

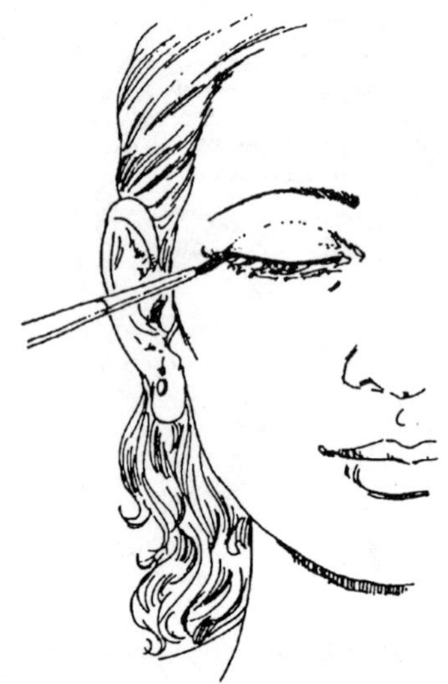

Fig. 13. Defining your eyes.

Use of eye pencils and kohl pencils: Pencils can be used in the same way to define or extend the shape of the eyes, but they give a softer, more natural line. Keep them sharpened and ready for use, as blunted or broken points can spoil the whole effect.

Mascara

Although eyeshadows define and dramatise your eyes, only your eyelashes are in a position to actually reflect colour into the eyes. So, to emphasise the colour of your eyes, you must frame them with an appropriate shade of mascara.

For the best result: First look down and brush the top lashes from the roots downwards (Fig.14A); then look up and brush the top lashes upwards (Fig.14B). Then still looking up, brush colour on the lower lashes (Fig.14C). Wait a minute for them to dry, and similarly apply a second

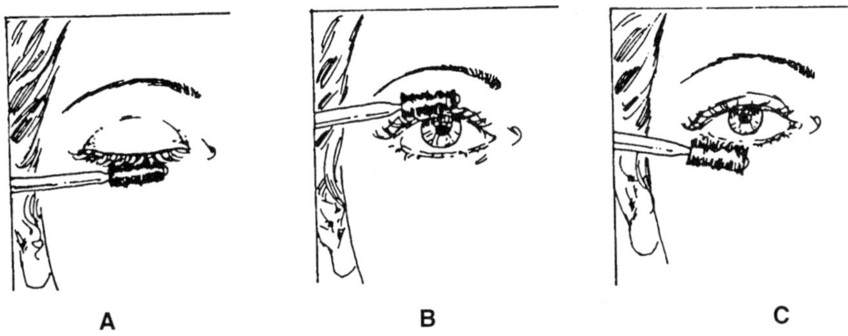

Fig. 14. Making the most of your lashes.

coat. Finally, brush with a clean dry brush to separate the lashes.

To remove the mascara: While removing the mascara avoid the colour from going onto the delicate area below the bottom lashes. Hold a tissue under the bottom lashes and close your eyes. Roll a cotton bud dipped in a cosmetic cleanser over the lashes, taking the mascara down onto the tissue. Repeat till all the mascara is gone.

Correction of eyes using make-up

You can improve your eye shape by experimenting with colour and texture. With some skilful shaping and shading, the eye can be made to look completely different. Identify the shape of your eyes and follow the tips given.

For small eyes: Pluck the eyebrows fine to give maximum eye area. Use a little shadow under the lower lashes as well as on the top of the lid. Blend the shadow on the upper lid from the centre outwards, curving it upwards towards the brow in the shape of a wing (Fig.15A). Line both the lids, extending the meeting line fairly out, to increase the length of the eyes. Mascara both the upper and lower lashes, using two coats on the outer lashes only.

For wide-set eyes: Pencil the eyebrows close to each other. Add a little shadow onto the bridge of the nose or blend your shadow close to the corner of the nose and stop at the centre of the upper lid (Fig.15B). To make the eyes appear a little closer, start outlining the upper lid from the inner corner of the eye, bringing it near the nose ridge, leaving just the width of one eye in between the two eyes. Continue the line towards the outer corner but not quite extending up to it.

For close-set eyes: Shape the eyebrows so that they don't have the close-together appearance. Use the eyeshadow on the upper outer half of the lid extending above the eye and under the brow (Fig.15C). To offset the closeness of the eyes, start drawing the eyeline on the upper lid away from the inner corner. Draw it up and out. Similarly, the lower line should not begin from the inner corner.

For deep-set eyes: Use a dark eyeshadow under the eyebrow, but not on the lid, where if you want to, you can use a lighter eyeshadow. Line only the lower lid and extend the line fairly out and up (Fig.15D).

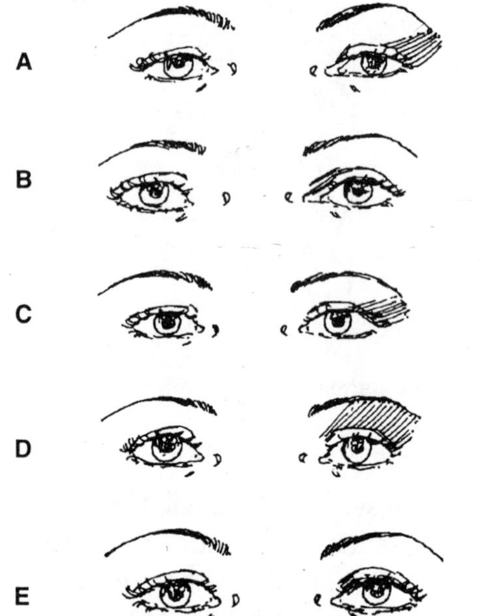

Fig. 15. Corrections of the eyes with make-up.

For round eyes: Make sure the shape of your eyebrows is angular. Blend your shadow from the centre of the lid and deepen it at the outer edge of the eye, extending it a little beyond the outer corner of the eye (Fig. 15E). Line the upper lids, starting from the inner corner and extend it out and up so as to suggest length.

Lipstick application

Lipstick provides the final touch to your make-up; without it no look is complete. For a perfect result, you will need a steady hand, some practice, the correct implements and knowledge of the correcting techniques.

What would you need? A narrow, flat ended brush, a selection of finely sharpened lip pencils, lipgloss and lipstick (either the conventional tube lipstick or the cream type with a sponge-tip applicator). If your lip colour is uneven, then you will need a special lip base or balancer – use a lighter tone on the dark areas and a dark tone on light areas. These balancers also form a base for lipstick and help to keep the colour of the lipstick pure and clear.

Application:

1. Outlining – Before outlining the lips, check that your lips are smooth and grease-free. Use a sharp pencil in a shade close to that of your lipstick colour and with a steady hand, lightly outline the lips. For the upper lip, start at the centre and work out, towards the corner of the mouth. For the lower lip, work from side to side (Fig.16A).
2. Priming the lips – Fill in the lips with a special base or balancer to even out the skin tones. If your lips are of an even colour, use a face powder as a base (Fig.16B).
3. Filling up – Using a lipstick brush, fill in the colour. For the upper lip, start at the centre and work outwards. On the lower lip work from side to side. Don't pile up too much colour. It is much easier to add more later than to remove any excess. (Fig.16C).
4. Blotting off – Fold a clean tissue and place it between your lips. Press the lips lightly together to remove the excess colour and to help seal the remainder, so that it stays on the lips rather than moving on to every glass you use (Fig.16D).
5. Finally finish with a lip gloss to get a gleaming look.

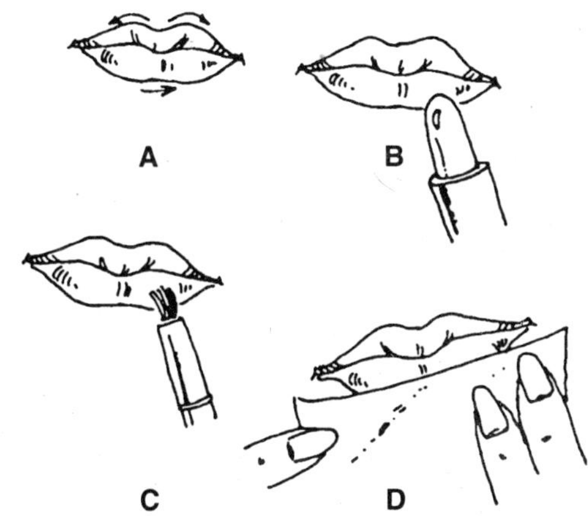

Fig. 16. Technique of lipstick application.

Shaping up

Through a knowledge of what you can do to correct lip shape you can truly achieve a perfect finish to your face. Study the shape of your lips, identify the defects, if any, and decide on what you want to achieve and then proceed.

For thin lips: These are easily corrected by taking the pencil outside the natural lip line (Fig.17A). Work slowly and steadily to form a perfect shape. Fill in with a primer and finally with the lipstick. A highlight of frosting on the upper lip would also create an impression of fullness.

For thick lips: These can be made to look smaller by drawing the outline just within the natural shape (Fig.17B). Use medium toned lip colours and avoid dark browns, plums, electric brights or pale shimmer shades.

For crooked lips: Asymmetry in lips should be studied well and you will be able to correct the shape by adjusting the outline to provide a perfect balance (Fig.17C).

For shapeless lips: Draw the most flattering shape by emphasising the centre of the upper lip and adding fullness to the lower lip (Fig.17D).

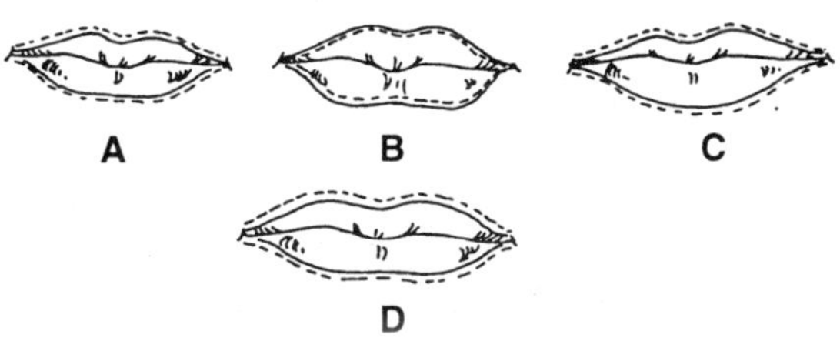

Fig. 17. Shaping up the lips.

Patching up

If make-up has to be touched up during the day, only powder make-up should be applied, using a brush. Use gentle patting strokes and blot the excess off.

●●●

3. Skin Diseases

DRY SKIN

What causes dry skin?

Normal healthy skin looks pink, feels smooth and soft and is well preserved. If the superficial skin cells are deprived of water, the skin looks parched and cracked, and feels rough and hard.

There are several reasons for developing dry skin. It can be a result of frequent washing (which removes natural oils) or a failure to protect the skin with regular applications of a moisturising cream. Certain environmental factors like wind, sun exposure, and overheated homes can also dehydrate the skin. Sometimes dryness is hereditary — then it is called *ichthyosis*. And as we age, our skin gradually becomes rough and parched.

Treatment to follow

Here are some suggestions which you will find useful, if you have a dry skin:

a) Use liberal amounts of oils and moisturisers. It is best to use these after a bath. Never apply the moisturiser or oil before a bath.

b) Avoid soaking in baths; showers are less drying.

c) Use rubber gloves while doing household chores.

d) Avoid getting your environment too dry, specially if you are used to air-conditioning.

e) Use cosmetics formulated especially for dry skin, because many other cosmetics may have a drying effect.

f) If all this does not help you, visit your dermatologist.

ACNE

All you have wanted to know about acne

Acne is one of the commonest skin problems. It produces unsightly spots on the face, neck, chest, back and upper arms. Although traditionally considered a teenage problem (8 out of 10 teenagers suffer from it!), acne can affect people even in their forties. One out of every 20 persons in the fourth decade has acne.

Even though it is a common problem, acne causes much anguish in the victims — so much advice is proffered to them that they really do not know what to do. Moreover, acne can sometimes go on for ages, producing both physical and psychological scars.

The sebaceous gland is the site of the problem — as mentioned earlier, these glands produce sebum which contains cholesterol, fatty acids and waxes. Several things can go wrong with this fairly simple process. For example, if the production of sebum increases or if dead cells clog up the openings of the glands, the flow of the sebum gets disturbed. The pores get blocked and blackheads and whiteheads form. Later, red, swollen and inflammed pimples develop as the sebum spills into the surrounding tissue. These pimples might even get infected.

Male hormones, the androgens, are thought to be responsible, at least in part, for the over-production of sebum and the consequent development of acne. In the past, diet had been held responsible for aggravating the problem. Hence for years, chocolates, spices and fatty foods were considered a taboo for acne patients. Recent studies, however, have scientifically exploded this myth. So, dietary restrictions are no longer necessary to combat the onslaught of acne.

Other factors which affect acne are menstruation, stressful conditions, hot humid climates and genetic factors. Cosmetic preparations containing lanolin and paraffin are known to exacerbate acne. Facial massage, often done to rejuvenate the facial skin, may actually result in acne. Pimples may also occasionally occur as a side-effect of drugs taken of other illnesses, like tuberculosis and fits.

A doctor's approach to acne

There is still a good deal of confusion about the best way to deal with acne — the confusion is constantly fuelled by the unbridled enthusiasm of some people who offer overnight cures. Don't get waylaid by such dubious claims.

Treatment can either be limited to the exclusive use of local applications or a combination of local treatment and oral medicines. As an important plank of local treatment, the importance of hygiene cannot be overemphasised. The simplest way is to wash the skin regularly and thoroughly with soap — this not only helps in improving the oily appearance, but also helps in reducing the occurrence of pimples. You can also use a slightly rough abrasive; this does not have to be anything special, a rough washcloth is good enough. Non-woven polyester webs have now been introduced and give excellent results. Greasy preparations for the scalp (oils) and face (creams, vaseline) should not be used. Many patients complain of an increase in pimples following facial cream massages — so these are best avoided.

Avoid squeezing your spots — this releases the gland contents into the tissues and so increases the inflammation. Some cosmetologists advise removal of blackheads – this is not only a time consuming procedure but is unlikely to reduce further appearance of acne.

Sulphur, the all important constituent of earlier acne treatments, is slowly giving way to newer drugs — *retinoic acid* and *benzoyl peroxide*. These cause scaling and redness of the skin but these side-effects are very necessary for the agents to be effective. These side-effects can be overcome by using newer preparations like adaplene. Locally applied antibiotics have been used to decrease the bacteria in the acne. *Erythromycin* lotion, and *clindamycin* preparations are effective anti-acne agents. Preparations containing *sodium lactate* or *azelaic acid* are also very effective.

Oral drugs are required when acne is moderately severe and cannot be controlled by local measures. Oral antibiotics then form the pivot of therapy; the most frequently used antibiotic is *tetracycline,* though *sulphas* and *erythromycin* can also be used. Despite prolonged use, say for six months to a year, no serious side-effects are usually associated with the use of *tetracyclines.*

Hormonal preparations have also been found useful in the treatment of acne. The *contraceptive* pill is used only if the patient has not improved with antibiotics treatment. *Anti-androgens* are also used sometimes. A note of caution is that these drugs should be used by women only, as they have unpleasant side-effects in men.

A drug, *isotretinoin,* has revolutionalised the treatment of acne, especially the severe variety. It is a derivative of vitamin A. Though expensive, the medicine holds hope for patients suffering from severe forms of acne. Scars which result from acne require specialised care and management. This aspect of acne is discussed later.

DISCOLOURATION OF SKIN

Leucoderma is curable

Leucoderma is an area of skin which has lost its colour. When it occurs without any preceding disease it is called vitiligo. Sometimes it follows burns and injuries. Some women develop it after the use of stick-on 'bindis' and after wearing plastic foot-wear — this loss of colour is due to chemicals present in the plastics.

Patches of leucoderma can be of variable sizes and shapes. They can occur just about anywhere on the body. In fair individuals, leucoderma often goes unnoticed, but on dark skinned people it can be very visible and cause severe embarrassment. Leucoderma does not cause any health problems — it is not contagious or dangerous at all. It is only a cosmetic problem.

There are a number of misconceptions regarding the availability of treatment for leucoderma. There is actually plenty of hope for vitiligo patients. The results with treatment are good. They are excellent if the treatment is taken early, but the patches of leucoderma which occur in areas of the skin which are naturally hairless, like the palms and soles, take long to improve.

Psoralens are the mainstay of treatment. These are nothing but purified form of *babchi* — the age old remedy. Pigmentation occurs with the help of sunlight. Both oral medicines and ointment form are available. A single small patch can be camouflaged using cosmetics. If the patches are extensive and generalised, then it would be simpler to get rid of the small amount of natural pigment present, so as to get a uniform colour for the whole body.

Role of surgery in leucoderma

Surgical techniques are not the first line of treatment for leucoderma. They should be used in patches of leucoderma resistant to medical therapy. Several methods are available:

- *Punch grafting*: In this, small cylindrical pieces from pigmented skin of the patient's body are grafted on the patch of leucoderma. It is then hoped that the pigment will spread from the grafted skin.
- *Melanocyte transfer*: Here the melanocytes are transferred onto the skin affected with leucoderma.

Darkening of skin

Pigmentation of the skin can be due to a variety of causes; the commonest is the darkening of the forehead, cheeks, and chin occurring in chloasma. Chloasma most often occurs in women during pregnancy or in those who are taking birth-control pills. It may sometimes also affect men.

The second type of pigmentation is freckling, a problem which is inherited. It is more commonly seen in fair individuals, particularly in those with red hair and blue eyes — so it is uncommon in our country. Both chloasma and freckling can be treated with bleaching agents like *hydro quinone*.

The third type of pigmentation is the darkening seen under the eyes — these are best managed by the clever use of cosmetics and by the use of under eye concealers.

Pigmentation of the skin can sometimes occur with hormonal disorders like thyroid disease or diseases of the adrenal hormones. The pigmentation in such cases is more generalised and may be associated with other symptoms. Such pigmentation needs to be investigated.

INFECTIONS

Boils

Boils are bacterial infections of the skin. They are very painful and if they appear in crops, they may be accompanied by fever. Some people have a tendency to develop boils. If you have been getting crops of boils repeatedly, it is worthwhile to get your blood sugar tested — your boils may well be a sign of diabetes.

The simplest remedy for a boil is to apply warm compresses — a piece of clean cloth dipped in warm water is sufficient. The boil is then likely to burst soon and the pain rapidly decreases. You must see your doctor if the boil doesn't come to a head within a couple of days (because it may need lancing), or if it is in a particularly tricky spot, such as on the buttocks, or if you get a crop of boils. The doctor may then have to prescribe antibiotics for you to quickly control the infection.

Fungal infections

Several species of fungi attack the human skin in a variety of ways. The marks of one type of fungal infections of the skin are ring-shaped, hence the common name, ringworm. Another type of fungus causes light-coloured spots on the skin — this is called pityriasis versicolor.

The groin is the site most commonly affected with ringworm. In women the waist, where the 'sari petticoat' is tied, is frequently involved. In children, ringworm can cause baldness of the scalp and this problem is quite contagious. On the feet, fungi cause athlete's foot — there is scaling, itching, and maceration in between the toes. Fungi can also affect the nails.

Fungal infections are easily treated. Ointments and lotions are used to treat small lesions. *Tolnaftate, clotrimazole, ecanozole* and *selenium sulphide* are very useful. A host of effective oral therapy are available for extensive lesions and to treat nail and hair infections – *griseofulvin, ketaconazole* and *terbinafine*. Do not treat your infection with just about anything available over the drug counter, as this may increase your problem -- consult your doctor.

Warts

Warts are a very common problem. At any one point, 10% of the population will have a wart or two on their bodies. Warts are caused by viruses — they are infectious and affect children most frequently. Most warts disappear spontaneously without any treatment. It is because of this that there are several claims of marvellous cures. You just have to listen to old wives' tales and you may well believe that it is possible to get rid of your warts by blowing on them nine times on a full-moon night, or by rubbing them with horses' tails. Many of the modern remedies are not really any better either. So only if the wart is inconvenient, or particularly embarrassing or painful or spreading rapidly, should it be removed. Otherwise I think, they are best left alone — in all probability, they would disappear with time without any scars.

Warts on the feet tend to be painful because they get trodden on. So these should be removed by your doctor; the small warts can be removed straightaway, but the large ones would need to be softened with some chemicals like *salicylic acid* before they are removed. The process of removal is slightly painful but the doctor is likely to give you anesthesia locally to make the area numb. Methods like cryotherapy and electric therapy are also available to treat warts. Laser therapy, though effective, is very expensive. No safe and effective oral medication is yet available for treatment of warts.

Cold sores

Cold sores occur most commonly on the lips, though they can develop on any part of the body. They are caused by a virus — Herpes simplex. In adults, this virus, sometimes, also affects the genitalia. This type of infection is spread by sexual intercourse and forms one of the many sexually transmitted diseases. The virus of cold sores generally lies dormant in the body, but can be activated by colds, (hence the name cold sores) fevers, stressful conditions, emotional upheavals or any serious illness. The first attack is usually severe but recurrences are less severe. Each attack lasts for a couple of days, but generally the attacks tend to become less frequent with time.

It is best to avoid intimate contact with an individual who is having an attack of herpes. There are some relief giving measures for acute attacks:

- Cold compresses or ice can relieve the pain.
- Ether compresses (to be given by a doctor) would hasten healing.

Acyclovir, though expensive, can give considerable relief to people getting recurrent attacks of herpes, especially in the genital area.

Scabies

Few diseases carry so much social stigma as scabies. Most people openly express resentment when they are told that their itching is due to scabies. Actually, anybody can get scabies — the disease is caused by a mite, *Sarcoptes scabiei.* It is a highly contagious disease.

Scabies is passed on from one person to another through intimate contact, infected bedding and clothes or by sharing a bed. The mite can live on the discarded clothes for a couple of days. After contact, it takes about 6 weeks for the itching to start. The itching is more severe at night. Soon a rash appears on the body — this rash is not seen on the face and is most prominent on the hands, the waist, the abdomen and on the genitalia.

When you go to your doctor with complaints of itching, he generally examines your hands very carefully — this is because he is looking to see if you have scabies. If you follow the directions given by the doctor carefully, scabies is easily treatable. The whole family is to be treated together, even if only one member has the problem. *Benzyl benzoate* or *gamma benzene hexachloride* are used — both are very effective, but can have side-effects. The new drug *permethrin* is very effective. Now an oral preparation *ivermectin* is available and it does away with the difficulty of applying the medication all over the body.

Leprosy is absolutely curable

This disease has always been associated with extreme social stigma since it is thought to be highly contagious and incurable. Both these notions are absolutely wrong and baseless. Leprosy is caused by a bacteria which is closely related to the germ of tuberculosis. It is the least contagious of all infections. If the treatment is taken early, it is easily cured; if, however, the treatment is delayed, then deformities develop; but even these can be corrected with surgery.

The most important symptoms of leprosy are decreased sensation and the appearance of light-coloured patches on the skin. The nerves might become painful. If the treatment is not taken at this stage, deformities might develop. Treatment of leprosy is available at all the hospitals. Nowadays, multiple drugs are used to ensure a total cure — *dapsone, clofazimine* and *rifampicin* are the drugs commonly used. Medication needs to be taken regularly for a duration varying from 6 months to 1 year. Interestingly, if the patient has only 1-2 patches of leprosy, the doctor may just give you a single day's therapy — in the doctors' jargon, this is called ROM (for the medicines in the pack). The medicines for treating leprosy are available in blister packs, free of charge, all over the country (and world!). Before starting the treatment, the doctor might take a piece of the skin to study it under the microscope — this will help him decide about the duration of treatment.

There are several myths about leprosy which need to be dispelled. For centuries, it has been perpetuated that leprosy is a curse. This is not true because it is just another infection caused by bacteria. It is also not an inherited problem and it cannot be transmitted from the mother to an unborn child. Leprosy is curable — even the deformities are amenable to surgery.

Complications of leprosy

There are a couple of complications which may occur in the course of leprosy:

- Due to loss of sensation, the patient may develop ulcers, which heal only very slowly.
- Weakness develops due to damage to nerves. This results in deformities.
- Reactions: These are acute exacerbations in the course of disease. The doctor might need to prescribe corticosteroids orally to prevent damage to nerves.

SKIN ALLERGIES

Causes of skin allergies

When the skin cannot tolerate certain substances, it reacts to their presence; this reaction can be either in the form of eczema or in the form of hives; this results in itching and redness of the skin.

It is often difficult to pinpoint the cause of allergy. It could be something you've ingested (foods, medicines, drinks) or something you've applied (cosmetics, antiseptics) or something you have worn (clothes, jewellery) or sometimes even something you have only touched (detergents, plants, vegetables, chemicals). So looking for the cause is sometimes really like looking for the proverbial needle in the haystack.

Deciding exactly what has caused the allergic reaction is difficult for several other reasons too:

1. The reaction may take a few hours to a few days to develop; it may not develop immediately.
2. Cosmetic companies are extremely secretive about the ingredients of their products, making it difficult for the patient and the doctor to identify the cause of the rash.
3. The reaction can develop even to minute amounts of the substance and the patient might not even be aware of the contact.
4. Moreover, the substance can get on to the skin in all sorts of indirect ways; for example, nail varnish can easily cause reactions on the face because we all touch our face several times a day.

Eczemas

Eczema is a rough red oozy rash that comes in patches. The fluid which has oozed then dries up to form a scab. Because the area is itchy, it often gets scratched and may become infected.

Eczema can develop in a number of ways:

1. Irritation of the skin can lead to eczema; the common causes are overexposure to water, soaps and detergents. Just about anyone can develop an irritant eczema, but the problem is much more common in people with dry skins.
2. Allergic reactions to substances which come in contact with the skin can also result in eczemas. This could

result from contact with metals (jewellery), vegetables, plants, and medicines.

3. Eczemas can also result from eating certain foods or taking certain medicines. Almost any food stuff can cause eczemas, but the ones that most commonly cause problems are eggs and dairy products.
4. Inherited eczema or what the doctor would call 'atopic eczema' is a problem seen most commonly in small children. The eczema tends to improve as the child grows up. It is less frequently seen in children who are breast-fed. Close relatives of children suffering from atopic eczema may have asthma or skin problems. A few of these children may also develop asthma when they grow up.

A few points to remember:

1. Eczemas are not contagious — don't shun a person with eczema; you are unlikely to contact it by touching such a person.
2. Some eczemas may recur — but most can be controlled with appropriate treatment with *steroid ointments* and anti-allergic medicines.
3. Keep your skin well hydrated; dry skin aggravates the problem.
4. Sweating makes eczema worse — so stay in a cool environment.
5. Direct contact with woollens and synthetics should be avoided as this aggravates the problems.

Hives or urticarias

Hives are temporary swellings of the skin, caused by a localised collection of fluid in the dermis due to leakage from the blood vessels. Urticaria can result from any of the following: (a) allergy to foods, pollens or drugs; (b) change in the temperature; (c) infections, including the presence of worms and (d) emotional upsets. Many times the cause cannot be accurately determined. A few individuals get hives repeatedly, but in most people urticaria usually gets better over a period of time.

If the cause can be made out, it is easy to cure urticaria. If the cause is not obvious, then a very effective way to get relief is to use anti-allergic drugs (antihistamines) for some weeks till the problem subsides.

Several antihistamines are available in the market. Many of these drugs cause drowsiness and slowing of reflexes and so the patient should not drive after having taken such anti-allergic drugs (hydroxyzine, diphenhydramine and chlorpheniranine). The newer antihistamines are either less sedating (cetrizine, loratadine) or non-sedating (fexofenadine). Remember to check the drug you have taken before you drive.

CARING FOR YOUR FEET AND HANDS

Problem feet

It seems that 9 out of 10 people have problems of the feet — cracked feet, fungal infections in between the toes, corns and ingrowing toe nails. It is really easy to prevent these problems — just a few precautions and you can have trouble-free feet.

Choose your shoes carefully and sensibly. Cut the toe nails regularly and, more important, carefully. Dry your feet well. The socks you wear should be clean. Air your feet well to prevent them from smelling and developing athlete's feet. Consult a specialist for corns — avoid self-help.

Dry skin of the feet can be improved by the regular use of creams, while hard skin can be kept at bay with the old-fashioned pumice stone. If you develop painful fissures, consult a doctor. These fissures are best treated using *salicylic acid* or urea ointments.

Choosing your shoes

Wearing shoes that really fit and provide the necessary support is very important. Wear the sort which grip and support your feet without cramping them. When buying shoes, always look at them from the following three points:

- Are they well made?
- Are they well designed?
- Do they fit well?

Remember that even a well-designed shoe must fit the foot. You can't hold the shoe in your hand and check its fitting — it must always be tried on the foot. Any shoe must be long and wide enough to allow the toes to lie flat. Check the fitting of the shoe at the heel too. The shoes should grip the heel and must support the full width of the heel. Moreover, the feet should not slip forward in the shoes. If the shoe is sloppy either in fitting or in design, then the only way it can be held on is by gripping downwards with the toes. This is not only tiring, but can also buckle the toes. The way the shoe is fastened is also very important — fastening two-thirds of the way up the instep is usually required to hold the foot back in the shoe.

Finally, make sure the shoe is stable and not too high-heeled. High heels are bad for your feet, because they throw your weight on the slender bones in the front. Also the foot then tends to slip forward, buckling the toes. High heels also affect the body's centre of balance, by putting strain on the parts of the body not designed to cope with it. The whole posture is affected and the muscles of the legs, pelvis and spine have to work much harder, and can get distorted.

Problem hands — a little care

Beautiful, smooth hands reveal a great deal about your personality. Well-cared hands are noticed and admired, even if they are not perfectly shaped.

Your hands are under constant assault by water, chemicals, vegetables, thorns, knives and what not. All these leave behind an indelible mark, unless you constantly look after the skin of your hands. This skin is tough — but not really that tough. So, it needs to be protected, otherwise it would become rough and dry.

You can prevent the roughness of your hands by using a good lubricating hand-cream. Coconut oil, vaseline and even the good old cooking oil are effective substitutes. Avoid immersing your hands in water for long periods of time because you are likely to develop infection of the skin around the nails (paronychia). You should wear rubber gloves while doing the household chores — these are really good for your hands and for your nails too.

Sometimes allergic reactions develop when you touch some objects like metals, plants and even vegetables, etc. If you know what is causing the problem you must avoid touching it. If you cannot recognise the culprit, gloves are a very useful way to protect your hands.

MOLES AND TUMOURS

How dangerous are moles?

Moles are actually an abnormal multiplication of the pigment cells of the skin. They are usually brown or black, but may sometimes be pink. They can be smooth or irregular, flat or raised and may even be hairy. They can be present absolutely anywhere on the body. Moles begin to appear in childhood and continue to increase during adolescence. An average adult has between 15-20 moles spread over the body.

Majority of the moles are entirely harmless. Rarely, however they become cancerous. For this reason, any mole which appears later in life or one which changes in size rapidly or one which has a tendency to bleed needs to be shown to the doctor. Ordinarily, moles are best left alone unless one is causing problems or is really unsightly. Removal, unless it is done carefully and by an expert, can leave behind ugly scars.

How serious is skin cancer?

There are a number of different types of skin cancers; some are very very slow growing and easily treatable, others spread rapidly and are difficult to treat.

Some facts about skin cancer you should know:

1. Skin cancer generally occurs either in areas which are frequently injured (like the foot) or on areas which are exposed to the sun (like the face).
2. Skin cancer is more common among the fair-skinned and in those parts of the world where there is plenty of sunshine.
3. It may develop in burn scars, and in old wounds.
4. It can develop in areas of the skin exposed to extremes of temperature, for instance, *kangri* cancer occurs on the part of the skin which is in contact with the *kangri*.

The treatment depends on the type of skin cancer and how much it has spread — the earlier the treatment started, the greater is the chance of a complete recovery. Skin cancer can often be cured permanently without any risk of recurrence. The different types of treatments available are — surgery, radiotherapy and anti-cancer drugs. Which treatment is to be used depends on the stage of the cancer and the type of cancer. Sometimes a combination of treatments is given.

AGE AND YOUR SKIN

Dealing with stretch marks

As a small child grows, his weight and height increases; so the skin has to stretch to accommodate this gradual, albeit massive increase in mass. At times, especially when there is a spurt in the growth, the growth of the skin fails to cope up with the growth of the body; the stretch then forces the elastic fibres in the skin to rupture, resulting in stretch marks or *striae*. These marks can develop at any time of life, but there are two occasions when they are particularly likely to develop:

1. During the adolescent growth spurt, about half of all children develop stretch marks. Marks usually show up in parts of the body where the elastic fibres of the skin are put under the greatest stress. Varying in length, they are pink to start with and invariably fade to white scars as years go by; they finally become wrinkled and papery and are then barely perceptible. Adolescent boys usually develop striae on their backs, buttocks and abdomen, while girls develop the marks on their breasts as well.
2. Women also develop stretch marks on the tummy and breasts during pregnancy.

Though there is no certain way to prevent stretch marks from developing, scores of preparations are available in the market, all claiming to do just this; many of these contain exotic additives like *collagen*, *vitamin A* and *allantoin*. These creams are as good as or as bad as plain moisturising creams in preventing stretch marks and nothing better. Gentle exercising of the abdominal muscles is suggested as a way to prevent stretch marks during pregnancy. Stretch marks on the breasts can be minimised by wearing a good maternity bra.

Once the marks have developed, the most effective way to deal with them is by using a camouflage cream. Most times, however, this is not required because these marks are on parts of the body which are generally covered. Many patients want to know about the efficacy of surgery. Surgery is definitely not advised, because the scars of surgery may eventually be more noticeable. Also although they rarely disappear entirely, stretch marks usually fade as years go by. So it is really best to leave stretch marks alone and allow time to be the true healer.

Skin changes and wrinkles

As we grow older, several changes become apparent on the skin:

1. There is a patchy increase in the amount of pigment in the skin; so eventually the skin appears blotchy.
2. Dead cells collect on the skin — this results in dryness and roughness of the skin.
3. The natural oil production is reduced, adding to the dryness of the skin.
4. The connective tissue beneath the skin loses its natural elasticity, because the elastic fibres break down.

All these changes combined with the effects of the different environmental factors like the sun, winds, and chemicals produce wrinkling of the skin. Smoking has often been mentioned as a reason for the early development of wrinkles. This is probably because smokers tend to screw up their eyes against smoke — the wrinkles then develop along these lines.

Although it is not possible to totally prevent the development of wrinkles, it is possible to slow down the process:

1. The sun is a giant wrinkling machine — so the simplest and the most

effective way would be to keep out of the sun and to use sunscreens if it is necessary to go out in the sun.

2. Using a good moisturising cream regularly reduces the dryness of the skin. For this you can use any moisturising cream — the fancy, expensive nourishing creams with exotic contents are actually no better than the ordinary creams. Though massaging the skin with creams is a frequently recommended advice, this suggestion is absolutely empirical. As a matter of fact, some dermatologists even believe that massaging may actually hasten the appearance of wrinkles.
3. Several medications have been found to retard sunlight-induced, wrinkling (photoaging):
   - Retinoic acid (0.025%, 0.05%), a frequently used antiacne agent, definitely reduces photoaging. It also reduces the blotchy pigmentation.
   - Hydroxyacids, like glycollic acid (10%).
4. Exercise is also often promoted as an effective way to stay young. Complex routines are designed to strengthen the facial muscles — but again there is no evidence that these exercises retard the development of wrinkles.

There are countless remedies available for wrinkles — most of them are actually useless. The popular anti-wrinkle creams are nothing but masking creams, they just camouflage wrinkles. Vitamin E enriched creams have been used extensively (with marginal effect!) Creams containing retinoic acid and glycollic acid may help. Special electric treatments and laser therapies are offered by beauty houses at exorbitant rates, though there seems to be little benefit from these and they may actually even harm the skin. Special diets and anti-wrinkle pills are also a waste of money. Vitamin supplements also do not help wrinkles. A simple and cheap way is to cleverly use make-up to camouflage the wrinkle lines — and this is what is most frequently used.

Surgery is the only definitely effective way of getting rid of wrinkles — there are several methods available but the best results are obtained with a face lift. This has been discussed in a separate chapter.

●●●

4. Hair and Scalp

The original function of hair was to keep the animal warm and afford protection. In certain animals it was also concerned with sexual and social communication (such as the mane of the lion). In humans however, hair tends to be primarily associated with the appearance we present to the world — it is a very convenient and yet a dramatic erotic signal: for a woman, beautiful hair is one of the most powerful weapons in her sexual armoury and for a man, it is the most visible sign of his virility.

Good looking hair is essentially healthy, shiny and clean. But our hair is constantly exposed to the aggressions of the environment and age and these tend to have a negative influence on its appearance — so most of the hair-care products we use, aim at reducing these effects, thereby making the hair look attractive as our crowning glory.

STRUCTURE OF HAIR

Hair is all protein

The part of the hair we see is dead; the actual living part is very small and is at the root in a part known as the papilla. In the papilla, cells multiply and produce a protein called *hard keratin* — this is responsible for the hardness of the hair.

The part of the hair which is within the skin, is enclosed by a sleeve of tissue called the *follicle*. Next to each follicle is a sebaceous gland, the oil producing factory of the skin. This oil forms a natural protective film over the length of hair, keeping it soft, shiny and supple.

Each hair is made up of three layers: the *cuticle* or the outermost layer, which has tiny overlapping transparent scales. When the scales lie flat against each other, the hair appears shiny, but when the scales are lifted, hair seems rough and dull. Conditioning rinses help to keep the scales positioned correctly, giving it a smooth and shiny appearance.

The cuticle of the hair is selectively porous. This porosity varies along the length of the hair, the youngest bit near the scalp being the least porous. Also oily hair is less porous than dry hair. The porous nature of hair allows for the penetration of chemicals. The agents used in bleaches, tints and perms capitalise on this nature of the hair - the chemicals used are quickly absorbed and bring about the necessary changes in colour and curliness.

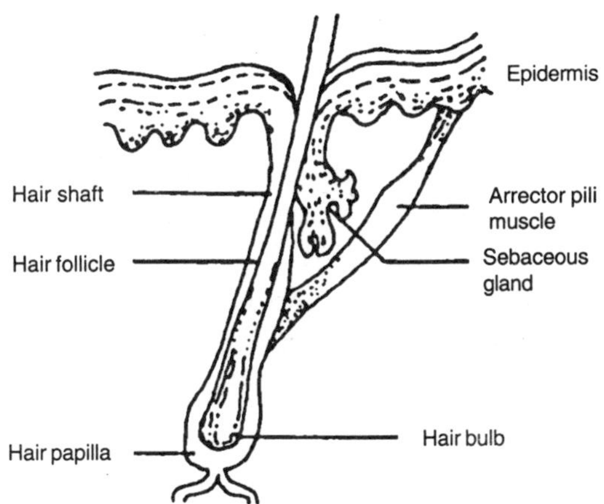

Fig. 18. The hair under the microscope

The *cortex* or middle layer of hair contains the colour pigment granules. The colour of hair depends on the number, size and distribution of the pigment granules in the cortex and also on the nature of pigment present. Colourants and bleaches work by penetrating the cuticle so that the colour is added to or subtracted from the cortex. The innermost layer is the *medulla*; it is absent in very fine hair.

SHAPE AND COLOUR OF HAIR

Straight hair or curly hair?

Curly hair has a flattened cross-section while straight hair has a circular one. The basic hair form is controlled by a number of genes - but this hair form is readily altered by chemicals present in perming and straightening lotions.

Thick hair or fine hair?

Except for palms, soles and lips, hair is present all over the body. In some areas, it is long, thick and dark – this is the terminal hair seen on the scalp, on the face of adults and in the axilla and pubic region of adults; some terminal hair are also present on the arms, legs and body. The hair on the rest of the skin is short, fine, light, and inconspicuous; this type of hair is called the vellus hair.

Sometimes hair which is normally supposed to be fine and inconspicuous becomes visible; for instance, terminal hair appears on the face of women in a condition called hirsutism. On the other hand, sometimes terminal hair gets converted into fine vellus hair – this happens in the all familiar baldness seen in men (androgenetic baldness).

Colour of your hair

The colour of your hair depends on the number, size and distribution of pigment granules in the cortex and the nature of the pigment present. The granules in black, blonde and red hair are different chemically; the brown black hair is due to *eumelanin*, the blonde hair contains *phaeomelanin* and red hair *erythromelanin*.

It is thought that a number of genes influence the colour of the hair – some of these genes also influence other inherited characteristics as well; the association between hair colour and hair form is well established. There is also an obvious association between hair colour and the colour of the eyes, the colour of the skin and the presence of freckles.

Though the basic colour of your hair is determined by your genes, this colour is readily altered by colouring agents. It can be lightened using bleaches, highlighted by a variety of agents and darkened by several types of natural and synthetic hair-dyes.

HAIR GROWTH

How fast does hair grow?

The rate of hair growth varies considerably but on an average it is one centimetre per month. The growth is greater in summer than in winter. It is maximum in the ages between 15 and 30 years. Cutting or shaving does not make hair grow faster. Neither does trimming affect the growth rate in any way (though trimming does make your hair look good by eliminating the straggly ends).

Each hair undergoes cyclic activity in three phases: the growth phase or *anagen* lasts for 3-4 years; following anagen is a short period of transition or *catagen*, following which is the phase of *telogen* or resting. During the resting phase (2–3 months) the hair becomes detached from its root and falls out, as a new growing hair replaces it in the follicle.

At a given time, 10-15% of the scalp hair are in an inactive phase, ready to fall out, while the remaining are in various stages of growth. A loss of up to 100 hairs per day is normal and is something you should not worry about as most of the lost hair would be replaced. With age, however, the rate of replacement slows down; so as you grow older, there is a natural tendency of some amount of sparseness of your scalp hair.

What controls the growth of hair?

1. *Family background and racial factors* are very important for the quality as well as the quantity of hair. Good quality long hair runs in families, and so does the all too familiar male types of baldness.
2. *Nutrition:* Hair, like any other aspect of your looks, is best improved by treating your system well. A good balanced diet is what is really required. An inadequate diet disturbs the structure, the growth and the colour of hair. When there is a total deficiency of protein, the hair becomes sparse, fine, brittle, dry, and light-coloured. The severe hair loss seen after crash diets is primarily due to protein deficiency. High protein diets, especially those containing gelatin and cysteine, increase the rate of hair growth. Deficiency of pantothenic acid leads to premature graying of hair in animals. Lack of essential fatty acids also causes hair to fall. Iron deficiency, especially in women, has been associated with hair loss, while iron supplementation hastens the growth of hair. Zinc deficiency also leads to hair fall. So an ideal diet for hair growth should contain adequate amounts of iron, zinc, protein and fatty acids.
3. *Age:* With increasing age, there is a decrease in hair growth. The replacement of shed hair is also incomplete and this results in sparsity of hair. In men, there is a recession of the hairline and sometimes definite areas of baldness appear. This baldness is dependent on the male sex hormones — the androgens. Rarely this hormone-mediated baldness is seen in women too.

4. *Hormones:* A number of other hormonal disorders can cause hair loss – thyroid disorders being the commonest. Though during pregnancy, hair loss slows down or may even stop altogether, excessive hair fall commonly occurs three to four months after delivery. Contraceptive pills also cause excessive hair loss and this stops when the pill is discontinued.
5. *Illness*: Any severe illness, be it physical illness (surgery, accident, fever, etc.) or even mental stress, can result in hair loss. However, this hair loss is reversible and recovers in about 3-6 months.
6. *Drugs*: Many drugs like anticancer medication can give rise to hair fall.

NORMAL CARE FOR YOUR HAIR

Which is better – combing or brushing?

If you use a soft brush, brushing is less damaging than combing, but a stiff brush does cause more damage to the hair than a comb. Prolonged brushing also harms the hair considerably. So the proverbial 100 strokes a night may actually harm the hair. Back-combing also damages the hair. It ruffles the scales of the cuticle as well as it causes knotting which is difficult to untangle.

Wet hair should never be combed or brushed because hair sticks together when wet and a greater force is required to comb or brush it and this causes greater damage to the hair. Moreover, the bonds (hydrogen bonds) which are responsible for the strength of the hair are broken temporarily when the hair is wet. This makes wet hair weak and more likely to be broken by combing or brushing.

A good comb should have rounded and not sharp teeth. Brush ends should always be rounded to minimise mechanical damage to the hair. Nylon brushes with spiky ends also damage the hair. The best hair brushes are made of bristles from the hair of wild boar; the tiny scales on the bristles clean the hair and give it a sheen.

How to choose your shampoo?

The aim of shampoos is not only to clean the hair, but to beautify it as well. Most shampoos are detergent based (lauryl sulphates). To this are added several chemicals — stabilisers, preservatives, conditioning agents, perfumes and colours.

A shampoo should be judged by its performance – not by its appearance, colour, perfume and definitely not by its price. It should clean the hair and rinse out easily, leaving the hair smooth and manageable. Lots of lather is not a measure of its efficiency – though it may indicate a high detergent content. Neither does a thick consistency mean that the shampoo is more concentrated.

There is a good range of products – labelled as 'for oily hair', 'for dry hair', and 'for normal hair'. The differences between these shampoos are in the type of the detergent used and also in the concentration of the detergent (being greatest for greasy hair) used. Shampoos with high detergent activity are based on anionic surfactants and those claiming mildness, generally contain non-ionic surfactants. Scientific studies have shown almost identical efficiencies for various shampoos, whether designated for oily or dry hair. All shampoos do leave behind a constant residue of oil because this is beyond the reach of surfactants – this is nature's way of protecting the hair fibres from injuries.

Regarding the pH of shampoos, it is generally agreed that neutral or slightly acidic shampoos are better for the hair; especially the hair that has been physically or chemically damaged. This is because the acids precipitate proteins on the hair surface which acts as a protective coat for the damaged hair.

How safe are shampoos?

Shampoos are very safe for the hair because they do not contain any harsh detergents, therefore the natural coating, the hydrolipidic film, is retained on the hair. Excessive cleansing may sometimes give rise to a 'flyway condition' of the hair. The hair then becomes unmanageable due to build up of static electricity. The main problem with shampooing, however, is the mechanical abrasion of wet hair caused by rubbing movements while shampooing and by towel drying. Reactions to shampoos are infrequent; the main problem is the irritation of eyes but the newer detergents and the chemicals in baby shampoos are free even from this problem.

How often should you wash your hair?

This depends on the type of hair and scalp, and also on the environment. If your hair is greasy then you would need to wash it frequently, say even 3-4 times every week. This is especially necessary, if the environment you work in is dirty. Frequent shampooing is not harmful to the hair.

Do exotic shampoo ingredients have any real effect on the hair?

Despite their popularity and appeal, many of the shampoo additives do not really benefit the hair, simply because they are quickly rinsed off the hair in the shampooing process. However some products, egg and beer for instance, may cling to the hair and impart apparent body to the hair and act as conditioning agents.

Some shampoos contain exotic, natural additives like collagen, gelatin, allantoin, and henna. Gelatin, which is nothing but the simplest of collagens, is almost ineffective. Broken down gelatin (hydrolysed gelatin) gives additional body and softness to the hair. Experiments have shown that it may be possible to even repair split ends, under optimal pH conditions, with hydrolysed gelatin. Amino acids and panthenol are added to some shampoos because they give body to the hair. Henna is another ingredient being used in more and more shampoos. The extract which is added is colourless and gives body and gloss to the hair without any colouration.

How do conditioners work?

There is nothing long lasting about the effect of conditioners – but they definitely do have a temporary magical effect on the hair.

Degradative changes of the hair are caused by combing, brushing, washing and drying. The scales of the hair cuticle are damaged – these then curl up and break. Since smooth overlapping scales are essential for shiny hair, the damaged hair appears dull and lifeless.

Conditioners do not penetrate the outer layer of the hair shaft – they merely coat the hair, helping to flatten and smoothen scales. A fine fatty film is deposited on the hair shaft; this temporarily fills in broken patches in the cuticle, just like plaster does over cracks in the wall. This softens the hair and gives it shine and body. Conditioners also restore the protective acidic film which is reduced during shampooing.

Hair is 'electrically charged' immediately after shampooing. So it easily tangles and becomes difficult to manage. The active ingredient of most *creme-rinse* conditioners is a cationic surfactant. This reduces the friction between hair fibres and increases surface conductivity, so the electric charge is lost and hair becomes manageable.

Which conditioner to choose?

Conditioners are generally used after shampooing. *Creme-rinses* are kneaded into the wet hair immediately after rinsing off the shampoo. The hair is then rinsed thoroughly after 1 to 2 minutes. If the conditioner is not rinsed off well, the hair may appear greasy.

Sometimes the conditioning agents are incorporated into shampoos; the conditioning performance of such combination shampoos is inferior to the performance of the 2-stage shampooing and conditioning. Newer conditioning agents (quaternary polymers) have, however, been added to shampoos without loss of the conditioning effect.

The term 'balsam' is frequently mentioned in connection with *creme-rinses*. The term is applied to conditioners which contain plenty of oils and protein. Exotic natural additives such as collagen, gelatin, allantoin and henna are also being used in the conditioners. Some of these have questionable effects while others add to the body and shine of the hair.

Are conditioners safe?

The conditioning compounds are not without adverse effects. The hair may be softened too much - this happens frequently with thin hair. A major problem with cationic agents is that they are highly irritating to the eyes and many cause defective vision due to the development of cataracts. As this happens with higher concentrations of the conditioning chemicals, their levels should be strictly controlled.

Home made rinses for your hair

Lime Juice, vinegar and tea water are often quoted as good hair rinses. They, in fact, do not offer the benefits of the easily available commercial conditioners. In the days when people used soap to wash their hair, a dull covering formed over the hair in the presence of hard water. All the above being acids, helped remove the soap scum. Nowadays this quality is of no value as the detergents used in modern shampoos do not precipitate with hard water. However, since most shampoos are alkaline, these acids do neutralise (weakly though!) the residual effects of the shampoos and may form an acidic coating on the hair.

INJURED HAIR

What is the cause of split ends?

If it is not cut, the hair can grow to a length of 40 to 80 cms. During its long stay on the scalp, the hair is exposed to innumerable physical and chemical traumas: combing and brushing, shampooing, weathering and chemical treatments. These factors are all the more damaging to hair because hair is a dead structure that lacks the power of self-repair. The cumulative effect of all these injuries is the gradual wearing down of the cuticle scales — these are totally lost at the tips of the hair and this results in split ends.

What can we do about split ends?

Though we cannot refrain from injuring our hair, careful grooming of the hair is likely to delay the appearance of 'splits': avoid rubber bands, spiky brushes and combs; avoid combing wet hair. Conditioners protect the hair against physical injury to some extent, so use them regularly. Once splits have appeared, it is a good idea to trim off the straggly ends to give a healthy appearance to the hair.

There is no definite way to mend split ends. Conditioners coat the hair and may temporarily bind splits, making them less obvious. Conditioning the hair with digested gelatin has been found useful. Singeing hair is a time consuming and a rather 'dare devil' technique which might 'singe off' splits but since it may even cause more damage to the hair, it is best not to be too adventurous.

Chemical treatment of hair

Chemical hair treatments include bleaching, oxidative dyeing, waving, and straightening of the hair. The integrity of the hair fibre depends on the presence of bonds (disulphide and ionic bonds) between various hair proteins. Chemical treatment of hair results in the breaking of the disulphide bonds, most of which are later reformed. However, even under the best of the conditions, 10 per cent of the broken disulphide bonds are not reformed, resulting in some residual weakness of the hair. So repeated procedures could eventually break the hair.

HAIR COLOURANTS

Hairdyes — natural and synthetic

The desire to mask the ageing process by hiding grey hair has existed throughout history. The hair colouring products which are available in the market fall into three main categories — the temporary colour rinses, the semi-permanent dyes, and permanent hair dyes. The various characteristics of the different types of hair dyes are given in Table 2. Of these, the permanent or oxidative hair colourants are the most versatile and most popular, despite their side-effects.

One commonly used hair dye is henna — a natural colourant. It is a permanent hair dye. Though henna imparts an orange-red colour to the hair, this colour can be altered by the addition of indigo logwood and camomile.

Table 2: Various characteristics of the different types of hair dyes

	Temporary colour rinses	Semi-permanent dyes	Permanent dyes
How they work	Water thin solutions or dispersions of certified dyes. Add a film of colour to outer cuticle; if damaged, some colour may reach and stick to the cortex. Hardly ever used.	Low molecular weight dyes. Penetrate cuticle to reach and adhere to cortex, without altering the structure of hair. Usually applied like shampoos with the lather left on for specified period and then rinsed off.	Have two ingredients that are mixed prior to the application: an oxidative dye precursor (para dyes particularly para-phenylenediamine) which determines the new colour and a developer which activates the dye precursor. Penetrate cuticle right into the cortical cells where they act chemically to change hair colour and structure. Most versatile of hair dyes. Very extensively used.
Effect of shampoo	Effect lasts only until the next shampoo when the cuticle scales open (due to effect of water on them) and colour molecules are washed out. Being water soluble, they are rain soluble too. May also rub off on linen etc.	Effect lasts between 4-6 shampooings, the colour fading gradually (the cortex is more absorbent and holds the colour for longer period).	Colour is not removed by shampooing, but remains until hair grows out or is cut off (because the colour molecules are fixed in the cortex cells). Subsequent dyeing is necessitated by the need to colour new hair growth and not due to fading of the already coloured hair.
Comments	1. Can produce subtle colour changes only. 2. Most effective on lighter hair. 3. Can temporarily blend.	1. Can produce noticeable colour change. 2. Can temporarily blend in grey.	1. Any colour change. 2. Patch and strand tests are necessary because para dyes are known to cause allergic skin rashes.

A real advantage with henna is that it is a superb conditioner. It gives the hair body and bounce. Moreover, allergic reactions to henna are extremely uncommon – all these advantages have made henna a favourite colourant specially with the 'nature product' faddists.

Hairdyes often cause reactions

Paraphenylenediamine is a major component of all the synthetic permanent hairdyes. It frequently causes allergic skin rashes – so it is necessary for you to do a 'patch test' before using these dyes, to check whether your skin is allergic to the hair dye.

For a patch test, prepare a small quantity of the dye. Apply it to the skin (usually behind the ear or on the inside of the arm, at the elbows) and leave it untouched and uncovered for at least 24 hours. The product should not be used for dyeing the hair, if any reaction (redness, irritation or blistering) develops. If there is no reaction, then it is safe to use the dye at that time. Since sensitivity can develop at any time (even after previous safe use), it is advisable to carry out a patch test every time you want to dye your hair.

Reactions to these dyes appear several hours after use. Although not very common, reactions, when they occur, are both painful and unsightly. Itchy swellings and oozing then develop on the scalp, neck, forehead, and eyelids. Some people also develop breathing difficulty soon after applying the hairdye.

Prolonged use of the hairdyes can result in the pigmentation of skin of the face and neck. Some doctors are of the opinion that hairdyes increase the risk of skin cancers – but this is really doubtful.

Hairdyes also weaken the hair protein and increase the porosity of the hair. This results in weakening of the hair. This weakened hair is more prone to other mechanical and chemical damage. Because of this effect, several permanent hairdyes available in the market incorporate conditioners into the dyes. These help to reduce the damage of the hair caused by hairdyes.

CURLING AND STRAIGHTENING OF HAIR

How do hair perms work?

Perming is a chemical process of changing the shape of hair, so that the new style is retained through several washes. Perming lotions contain chemicals which break some of the bonds within the protein fibres of the hair. The lotions remain on the hair for the necessary development during the period in which the desired number of bonds (25-30%) are broken. A new pattern is then imposed on the hair by winding it on rollers. The lotion is then rinsed off the hair and a neutraliser is applied to enable the disrupted bonds to reform with a new pattern, giving the hair a new shape.

Perming can be achieved either by a cold process or by a hot process. In cold waving, thioglycollates are used to break the bonds, while in hot waving, alkalis are used. 'Soft perms' are also available for home use – they act in the same way but contain bisulphites which act more slowly and to a lesser extent – the result is a softer perm which does not last very long. Normally the professionally given perms should last until the treated hair grows out or is cut off.

What can go wrong with a perm?

A number of factors combine to make the perm successful: the correct strength of the lotion, the curler size, the degree of tension with which the hair is wound around the curlers, and the development time. Things can go wrong with any of these and spoil the perm.

You might not be satisfied with the style of the perm. With small curlers and too much tension on the hair, the hair looks frizzy. Similarly, in case of too long a development time the curl becomes too tight. With a short development time and larger curlers the perm is loose.

Damage to the hair is another problem with perming; this occurs most often in the hair which is already damaged by dyeing. Even in normal hair, too prolonged an application or too strong a lotion may cause damage, because of the weakening of the bonds in the hair protein. The cuticular scales are also damaged during perming and may even be lost — this leaves areas of hair naked making it look lifeless. If sufficient damage has been caused to the hair, it may break, either immediately or within a few days of perming, as you comb or brush your hair.

In rare cases, skin irritation can occur — this is the result of careless application of the lotion or if the lotion is allowed to remain for too long in contact with the scalp. In view of the problems your skin and hair are likely to face, it is better to get your hair permed from an experienced beautician.

How often can you perm your hair?

This depends on the condition of your hair. Some damage does take place during perming and this is more so if the hair has been dyed earlier and it is therefore better to avoid re-perming your hair earlier than 4-5 months.

Can curly hair be straightened?

Yes, hair can be straightened just as it can be curled. This is done either by using chemicals or heat. The hair straightening is brought about by breakage of the bonds and formation of new ones and this too makes the hair weak. Of the chemical methods, one technique uses a strong alkali and the other involves the use of a reducing agent. The former tends to have a stronger effect.

SETTING YOUR HAIR

What are setting agents and hair sprays?

Setting agents keep the hair set longer. They are applied to the washed hair before it is set. A film of the agent is left on the hair and as the hair dries, it is glued together giving it a stiff and thick appearance. Hair sprays, on the other hand, are used on hair which has been set. They keep hair in place.

Both, setting agents and hair sprays have very little chemical effect on the hair proteins. They both contain water soluble polymers, but in different formulations. Mechanically, they have two different effects: because they minimize the need to comb, they reduce hair damage; but they make hair stiffer, so it becomes difficult to comb, thereby increasing the damage to the hair while combing. Both these opposing effects are generally balanced.

Blow drying

Many of us use a 'dryer' for setting hair. Sometimes we use it simply to rapidly dry wet hair. Heat is potentially damaging to the hair because it results in the loss of natural oils and moisture. Also 'heat treated' hair is more prone to damage, because heat weakens the hair protein. This is especially so if the hair was wet prior to heat drying.

It is best to avoid a dryer altogether; but if this is not possible, follow these precautions:

- Use the dryer when the hair is comparatively dry.
- Be gentle.
- Use a warm/cool setting on the dryer and keep moving it, so that no one section of hair is subjected to heat for too long.
- Don't hold the dryer too near your head.
- Direct the warm air along the direction of hair growth, so that you are blowing flat on the scales of each hair shaft and not ruffling them up.

●●●

5. Problems with the Hair and Scalp

ITCHY SCALP

If your scalp is itching, look carefully for lice

You might be surprised, but this pest has no respect for your social status. Apart from affecting the scalp, lice can reside on the body and on the clothes as well.

The lice suck blood from the skin and may cause infection. The main problem, however, is itching. The thing to look for, to confirm the presence of lice, are the eggs (nits) laid by lice; these are attached to the hair and are the size of a pinhead, so you really have to search carefully for them. Once the diagnosis is made, the problem is easily treated with *permethrin, malathion* or *gamma benzene hexachloride*; *permethrin* needs to be applied only for twenty minutes. It can be incorporated into shampoos, which are kept in contact with scalp for 15-20 minutes, and then rinsed off. *Malathion* and *gamma benzene hexachloride* are used overnight, once a week for 2 weeks.

What causes dandruff?

We all shed dead skin cells as a normal process; these cells are not shed off individually but as aggregates which are normally too small to be seen. In dandruff, however, the shedding of the dead cells is in larger visible aggregates; there is also an excessive production of dead cells. What causes this is not conclusively known — but it is definite that dandruff is not infectious. You cannot catch dandruff, just by using the comb of a person who has this problem.

Dandruff is rare in children. Scaling generally begins to emerge at adolescence. Starting at puberty, dandruff increases gradually over the next few years; it is maximum in the early twenties. Later over the years, it gradually decreases and is rare in the elderly.

Earlier, skin care people made a distinction between oily and dry dandruff. Today this opinion is held as absurd. Scientific studies have shown that the oil production in scalps with dandruff is the same as that of scalps without dandruff. Moreover, artificially degreasing the scalp does not decrease the amount of dandruff produced, even though the oiliness is decidedly reduced.

Getting rid of dandruff

There are two ways of treating dandruff: either the scales are removed as quickly as they are formed, or the formation of scales is suppressed. Shampooing is a good way to rapidly remove the scales. To be effective, the washing should be thorough and frequent. Application of oils temporarily improves the appearance of a scaly scalp because the scales stick to the scalp and are less visible. But oils tend to nullify the effect of shampooing to a considerable extent and are best avoided if you are suffering from dandruff.

Medicated shampoos are very popular; these may contain *selenium sulphide, zinc pyrithione* or *coaltar.* These agents decrease the production of scales in addition to removing the scales. *Corticosteroid* applications are also very effective in reducing the production of scales and are used for severe dandruff. But the most important aspect of treating dandruff is that the medications should be used regularly till you outgrow the problem.

GREYING OF HAIR

What causes greying of hair?

The colour of the hair depends on the presence of pigment granules in the cortex of the hair. With age, there is a gradual dilution of pigment in the hairs, so that in different hairs the full range of colours from normal to white can be found. The age of onset of this greying process is largely determined by your genes. The first evidence of grey hair usually appears in the third decade. Generally by the age of 50, 50% of the population have at least 50% grey hair.

Grey hair can sometimes appear earlier too. Premature greying of hair runs in certain families. Rapid greying of hair may occur after severe emotional stress. In certain internal diseases, hair might grey early. This is especially true of diseases of the thyroid gland and certain types of anaemias. Localised patches of grey hair can appear on areas of leucoderma.

What can be done?

The usual and the most effective way of dealing with greying of hair is dyeing it. There are several types of dyes available (these have been already discussed). The oxidative dyes are the most versatile and most frequently used, despite the fact that they can cause reactions. Henna is also used because apart from its safety, it is a superb conditioner.

Several patients of premature greying of hair have responded to *calcium pantothenate* in the dose of 200mg daily. So this form of treatment could be tried in children and in young adults.

DEALING WITH SUPERFLUOUS HAIR

Hirsutism and its causes

Most, if not all, adult males have visible hair growing on their faces and body. Women, on the other hand, have only very fine downy, inconspicuous hair on the face and body. If this hair becomes darker, thicker and visible, then the woman is suffering from hirsutism. This problem may cause intense misery and make the woman feel less feminine. They might even feel a bit of a freak. But, it must be remembered that unwanted hair especially on the legs, is actually present in as many as 6 out of 10 women.

The basic problem in hirsutism is the excessive action of the male sex hormones – the *androgens*. Increased amounts of androgens may be produced; for instance, tumours of the ovaries may be responsible for this. The blood levels of the androgens are then raised above normal. In most women with hirsutism, however, the androgen production is not increased. In them, because the normal downy hair are very sensitive to the low levels of androgens they get converted into thicker and longer hair.

Heredity and ethnic origin have a lot to do with the amount of hairiness of the skin. Mental tension and some medicines can also cause hairy problems. Women with hirsutism are often over-weight and infertile. They often develop severe acne on the face and frequently have sparse scalp hair. Rarely frank baldness, quite like that seen in men, develops. Infrequently, they develop frank masculinisation. So hirsutism may well be more than a cosmetic problem. So, if you are having hair problems, do consult your doctor.

Mild hirsutism may be a normal growing-up process; a few abnormal hair may appear at puberty or at menopause. However, a rapidly progressive problem or an association with infertility, definitely requires specialised types of investigations and treatment; in these patients just removal of the hair would be a totally inadequate solution, because the hair would rapidly grow back.

Can medicines help reduce hair-iness?

Treatment of hirsutism depends on the cause as well as on its severity. The cause needs to be determined by examination and investigations. Most often, simple investigations like X-rays and ultrasound examination of pelvis is sufficient. However, sometimes specialised investigations like estimations of blood levels of androgens, specialised X-rays and even a laparoscopy (visualisation of abdominal organs using a tube) may be required.

After the cause is established, it needs to be treated; a tumour will need surgical treatment. If the androgen levels are raised and sometimes even with normal levels of androgen, anti-androgens have been found effective. Anti-androgens are a new group of drugs which counter the effect of androgens. Three drugs have found use – *cyproterone acetate, spironolactone* and *cimetidine*. They are most effective when used along with cosmetic treatment of hirsutism; the hair regrowth is reduced and the hair which reappears is much finer, and finally over continued treatment, the hair becomes inconspicuous.

What can be done for superfluous hair cosmetically?

Hairy legs may upset one girl but not cause a shadow of worry in another. How much of the problem you have depends not only on the colour of the hair, but also on your state of mind. It helps to realise that there are many who have similar problems.

What you can do about it depends on the time and money you want to spend and more importantly by how much the problem is bothering you. If the hirsutism is mild, then camouflaging the hair is the best solution. In moderately severe varieties it may be necessary to remove the hair; this can be done by depilation or epilation. Depilation removes the hair at skin level — sometimes just below skin level. Epilation, on the other hand, removes the full length of hair.

Bleaching superfluous hair: Bleaching is one way of making existing hair less conspicuous — it is good for down, rather than for thick coarse hairs. It is the most commonly used method for camouflaging facial hair.

A simple bleaching system consists of hydrogen peroxide containing ammonia to give a pH of 9 to 10. There are several recipes for a home bleach — 2 teaspoons of fuller's earth mixed to a paste with one teaspoon of 20 volumes peroxide and six drops of ammonia. Apply the paste and leave it on for 5-10 minutes. Fancy packages of cream bleaches are now available, making bleaching very simple.

The only problem with bleaching is irritation. This happens either when too much ammonia has been added to the system or when the bleach is kept on for long periods. The reaction usually subsides after a few hours. When the reaction is mild it may help to apply a cream like *eumosone* or *sofradex* to reduce the redness. When the reaction is severe, a doctor's help should be sought.

Shaving does not make hair grow faster: It is a total fallacy that hair grows faster and becomes coarser after shaving. Yes, after shaving hair does reappear with great rapidity (within 24 hours) but this is not because hair growth has been stimulated, but because shaving cuts the hair just at the surface. Coarseness is apparent, because the hair is left with blunt tips. So shaving is an unacceptable method of dealing with facial hair in women, but is one of the most commonly used methods of dealing with superfluous hair on the legs and under-arms.

A further possible disadvantage with shaving is the risk of nicking the skin. This can be reduced by using a swivel head razor and shaving slowly and carefully. For best results, the razor blade must be sharp. Electric razors, though initially expensive, are a worthwhile investment. Wetting the hair makes shaving easier, as this makes the hair softer and more pliable. Applying soap keeps the hair wet for longer periods (but you must use an electric razor on absolutely dry hair). Avoid using an anti-perspirant or a deodorant for at least 12 hours after shaving.

You can use pumice stone to remove hair: Abrasives, in the form of pumice stones and special emery-covered mitts and pads are frequently used to remove unwanted hair. Though this method is very cheap, its effects are very temporary. But it is a good alternative for skins which tend to suffer reaction to other methods, provided you are gentle. If the skin is rubbed too vigorously, it will become tender and sore; so use gentle, circular movements and apply a moisturising cream after the use of abrasives. This method is most effectively used on moderately coarse hair of the legs and arms and is not practical for use on the face. After waxing, the regular use of pumice stone can delay the reappearance of hair.

Problems with chemical depilation: Depilation is the method commonly used for removing superfluous hair on the arms, legs and underarms; occasionally it is employed for removing facial hair – now specialised preparations are available for exclusive use on the face.

Depilatories are generally thioglycollate based and occasionally sulphide based. They weaken the hair protein, keratin, by reduction and hydrolysis in an alkaline pH (provided by calcium or sodium hydroxide). The hair breaks just below the skin surface. The time required for depilation depends on the coarseness of hair, varying between 5-20 minutes. Use of soluble alkalis, like sodium hydroxide, reduces the depilation time.

Depilatory agents are available as creams, lotions and sprays. Lotions are easier to apply over larger areas. Aerosol sprays are the latest methods of applying depilatories. They are quicker and more convenient, but need to be used carefully to avoid misdirection of the spray.

Irritation and dryness of the skin may occur, because the chemicals act on the keratin of the skin as well. This problem is usually minimal, because of the short time of contact. However, if the depilatory is reapplied immediately after the first application, irritation can occur. Dryness of the skin becomes evident after 24 hours. To counter the dryness, two stage products have appeared in the market; the second stage emollient soothens the skin and enhances the smoothness of the skin. It is buffered at acidic pH to ensure the neutralisation of any residual alkali. A similar effect can be achieved by swabbing the area with a neutralising solution, of 1 part lemon juice or vinegar to 7 parts of cold water, immediately after the depilatory cream has been removed and following this with application of cold cream.

Depilatories should never be used on broken skin. Since allergic reactions sometimes develop to depilatory agents, patch-testing should always be done before applying the chemicals on larger areas and if a reaction develops at the site of the patch test, the depilatory should not be used.

Waxing away hair: Waxing is one of the oldest methods of removing hair. Though the whole length of the hair is removed, it regrows because the hair papilla is not destroyed. Frequent waxing, however, does result in less conspicuous hair growth, because eventually the hair root does give up this unequal struggle and goes out of the business of multiplying.

Waxing is the method of hair removal most often used in beauty parlours, where beauticians heat pans of wax, judge the right temperature (not too hot and not too cold) and apply it in strips and rip it off quickly, taking the hair off with the wax. It sounds horrible but women do get used to it with time. Cold wax is the 'do it yourself' alternative, but it is inferior and also more painful than the hot wax method.

Waxing is a very popular method of dealing with unsightly hair on the legs, arms, and underarms. Repeated waxing does lead to finer growth. Moreover, there is no stubble, as the hair which reappears has tapered tips and the hair does not become obvious for about 3-4 weeks. The real problem with waxing is that one has to wait for a proper regrowth, for repeating the job and this may take a couple of months. The skin may appear a little angry for the first 12 hours after waxing. If not applied carefully, and if the wax is too hot it may cause burns. To overcome the angry look after waxing it may be useful to apply medicated creams like *eumosone* or *sofradex* soon after waxing. At around 2-3 weeks after waxing, some women develop a pimple-like eruption. This again can be prevented by using *sofradex* or *retinoic acid.*

Plucking and threading of hair: Plucking and threading are usually reserved for eyebrows, hairs on the upper lip and chin and for removing odd hair around the nipples. These methods do not increase the hair growth.

Plucking can be a rather painful process; it may help to wipe the area first with an ice cube to numb the nerve endings. But if you are threading, the wet hair will cling to the skin, making it difficult for you to thread; so for threading, it is best to lightly apply talcum powder to the area to separate the hair.

Getting rid of superfluous hair permanently — Electrolysis

Yes. Electric epilation is considered a safe and a cosmetically acceptable method of removing unwanted hair permanently. It is a useful way of getting rid of facial hair, but for hairy legs and arms it might prove too expensive and too time-consuming. Though X-rays, in sufficient dose, can also cause permanent epilation, their use for this purpose should be condemned because they have several dangerous side-effects.

Electric epilation may be affected by direct current of low voltage or by alternating current of higher voltage. Though the term 'electrolysis' has actually been loosely used to describe several methods of electric epilation, scientifically speaking, it should be applied only to the method of destruction of the hair-root by direct-current. Epilation by alternate current should be termed diathermy epilation.

In diathermy epilation, the tissue resists the passage of high frequency oscillations and the heat which is thus produced, destroys the hair follicle. Electrolysis is the less commonly used method today. In this method, the direct-current (galvanic current) causes chemical decomposition and death of the hair root.

How is electric epilation done? In both methods, a needle electrode is introduced into the hair-pore until resistance is encountered — this happens when the bottom of the follicle is reached. The current is then passed. If the papilla is destroyed, the hair can be pulled out easily with the fingernails or with forceps. If the hair does not come out easily, one or more additional short current applications are made and the hair is then removed.

New innovations have made electric epilation relatively easy. A unique hand-held galvanic epilator for electrolysis —

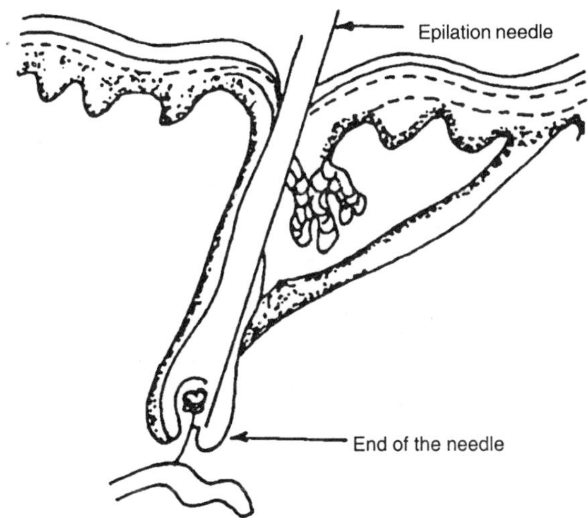

Fig. 19. Getting rid of superfluous hair permanently.

Perma Tweez, is now available for self-epilation. Sophisticated automatically timed diathermy epilators are useful when extensive areas have to be epilated. Some of the newer epilators even use sound and light waves.

Is electric epilation really safe? Both electrolysis and diathermy epilation, when performed by skilled, experienced and above all, qualified operators, are perfectly safe methods for removing unwanted hair. Home electrolysis devices are now available – but because it is so easy for the process to go wrong in unqualified hands, it is sincerely advised that you should seek professional help for electric epilation.

Does it hurt? That depends on the individual's pain threshold but usually the pain is bearable. In very sensitive women, pain can be greatly reduced by using a local anaesthetic to deaden the area. Using short bursts of current also makes epilation almost painless.

Removal of hair by electrolysis is safer and less likely to cause scarring. Ideally, the highest concentration of current should be located at the point where destruction is desired; if the current flows extravagantly, a cone of destruction occurs and this results in scarring. A bulbous tipped insulated probe has been developed to eliminate the leakage of current along the length of the needle. Short bursts of current tend to limit the damage. To lessen chances of tissue damage, contiguous hairs must never be removed. Despite all precautions, certain individuals would eventually develop scars; these people should absolutely avoid electrolysis. Scarring is generally in the form of small pits though sometimes hypertrophic scars appear – these are common in women who have a natural tendency to scar.

A practical problem with epilation is the time taken for hair removal. The number of hairs which can be removed at one sitting depends on the site of epilation, the type of hair growth and the experience of the operator. Diathermy epilation is faster than electrolysis and normally 75-100 hairs can be removed in a sitting of 15-20 minutes. So trained personnel prefer to use diathermy epilation.

Another problem with electric epilation is the regrowth of hair; following diathermy epilation, even in the best of hands, 20-30% of hairs which have been removed, grow back. In electrolysis, though the percentage of hair regrowth is much less, the hair which regrows is thicker than that after diathermy. So, on the whole, the patient is happier with diathermy epilation than with electrolysis because immediate results are more impressive. A newer innovation, with a bulbous probe, is termed *thermolysis*. This has a regrowth of only 5% and the scarring is much less and has truly been found very effective in treatment of hirsutism.

After treatment, the skin should be kept dry and an antiseptic cream used. In between sessions, it is better to avoid plucking or waxing the hair, so that when you go for electrolysis, the hairs to be removed are visible.

Laser hair removal

Laser hair removal is based on the fact that hair is the only pigmented structure in the dermis. It is important to remember that lasers can be used only to remove black/ pigmented hair and not grey hair.

Lasers which can be used: Not all lasers can be used for removal of hair. The 3 lasers which have been used for hair removal are:

- Ruby laser
- Diode laser
- Alexandrite laser

Usefulness of laser hair removal: Laser hair removal is a new technique and has not been studied extensively in pigmented skin like ours. In fair skin individuals, laser hair removal is safe and associated with minimal side-effects. In pigmented skin the skin may blister and heal with change of skin colour. However, lasers may offer the advantage of being less labour intensive and much faster.

LOSING HAIR

Baldness — What are the causes of excessive hair loss?

All of us lose hair. A loss of up to 100 hairs a day is normal, as this hair loss is replaced. Excessive hair loss which is not replaced leads to baldness.

Baldness or *alopecia*, as your doctor would call it, has several causes:

1. The commonest form is the baldness that affects men. It is called male pattern baldness. The hair loss in this condition depends on two factors, namely the presence of male sex hormones (the androgens) and a genetic tendency to develop baldness. One out of every ten men is likely to develop some degree of alopecia by the age of 25; by the age of 35, four out of ten men suffer from baldness; and by the age of 50, nearly half of all men are bald!

   The age of onset and the pattern of baldness and the rate at which it will progress are all inherited. Generally speaking, the sooner the baldness starts the more severe it is likely to be; so if a person has got a pretty good head of hair at the age of 35, he is very likely to keep it for a good many years more.

   Androgen dependent baldness can also occur in women. Small amounts of androgens are normally present in all women. If you have a very strong family background of male type of baldness, then your hair is probably very sensitive to even the low levels of androgens normally present in women. However, the pattern of hair loss in women is totally different. In them, hair is lost from the whole scalp and they do not generally develop obvious baldness. Acne and hirsutism may be associated with this pattern of baldness in women.

2. Many systemic diseases can cause diffuse hair loss. Any prolonged debilitation (typhoid, viral fevers, malaria, operations, accidents and even child-birth) can be followed by diffuse loss of hair. Mental stress must be included as a cause of this type of baldness – it can cause severe forms of alopecia. Hair begins to fall about 3-4 months after the illness and continues for about 3-4 weeks. Most of the hair which is shed, however, regrows in about 3 months.

   Nutritional deficiencies, crash dieting and anorexia nervosa are all associated with hair loss. Anaemia is an important cause of hair loss in women. Hormonal disorders, especially thyroid diseases and diseases of the ovaries are often associated with hair loss. Some medicines like contraceptive pills and anti cancer drugs can also cause alopecia.

3. The third type of baldness is called *alopecia areata*. Patches of baldness first appear on the scalp, but can spread to the eyebrows and eyelashes as well. In men the beard area may be involved. The patches develop rather suddenly and may be precipitated by stress. Fortunately, most of the time, the problem resolves on its own – the hair begins to regrow spontaneously within a few months. This pattern of alopecia is more commonly seen in men and is sometimes associated with leucoderma and diabetes.

4. Some diseases of the scalp can also cause baldness. Many people think that dandruff causes hair loss, but this is not true. In children, fungal infection commonly leads to hair loss. Sometimes, bacterial infections can cause baldness.

5. Finally physical trauma also results in hair loss; this type of hair loss affects women more often than it affects men. Tight hair styles, like ponytails for instance, literally pull the hair out by the roots. Baldness usually appears in the front of the scalp and improves, once the hair style is changed for a looser one. Using hair brushes with stiff nylon bristles can also cause baldness, as also using combs with tough teeth. Too much exposure to hot air can cause similar problems too, so you must use a hairdryer with care.

What is the remedy for baldness?

Baldness is an embarrassing problem and there is no treatment for several types of alopecias. So a huge range of commercial remedies claiming to increase hair growth have appeared in the market. Whether anything will help, depends largely on the cause of the baldness. There are no magic cures and a good many of the products available are absolutely useless. Many of the preparations sold for the treatment of hair loss are advertised with accompanying photographs showing before and after treatment pictures. These look very convincing, but if an individual with alopecia areata uses a hair restorer and improves, the restorer gets the credit when in fact the hair growth might well have begun spontaneously. Similarly, hair which is lost after prolonged illness will regrow without the help of any medicines.

What you can do, if you are suffering from baldness, is to make sure that any causative factor is dealt with. Consult your skin specialist for this and if he finds a cause for your alopecia, he would treat it and your hair would regrow.

Male pattern alopecia is one type of baldness which is difficult to treat. Even in this, now treatment is encouraging, though it may be expensive.

1. The easiest and the cheapest solution is to grow the remaining hair, and then to restyle it to cover the bald areas. Conditioning the hair would give body to the hair; but these methods can be resorted to only in mild cases of baldness.
2. A new drug, *minoxidil,* is now available to give relief to many balding scalps. A real problem with minoxidil is the high cost of the medicine. Also the hair growth is temporary; if you stop applying minoxidil, the baldness will come back.
3. Now, we also have oral medications available to treat this form of baldness – a drug by the name of *finasteride* can be taken in the dose of 1 mg daily. This drug, however, should be taken under strict supervision because it can cause temporary side effects like sexual dysfunction.
4. Another rather expensive solution to this problem is hair transplantation. It is based on the fact that hair, when transplanted from a hair producing area to a bald area of the scalp, continues to function and grow normally for a lifetime. If done with skill, this method seems to work fairly well.

●●●

6. Nail and Nail Care

Good nails are essential to natural beauty. Dry, bitten off, cracked nails really detract from the beauty of your hands and feet. By caring for the nails, you would be enhancing the appearance of your hands and feet. Just a few minutes of care everyday and a few precautions is all that is needed to make your hands and feet look smashing.

NAIL FORMATION AND GROWTH

How is nail formed?

To understand how best to care for your nails, you should know the structure of the nail and how it is formed. The part of the nail which is visible is called the nail-plate (Fig. 20). It is composed largely of a protein, *hard keratin*, which is very similar to the protein of the hair. On three sides, the nail-plate is covered by the *nail-folds*. It rests on the *nail-bed*, being formed at the base of the nail-bed in the part called the *nail-matrix*; the nail-matrix is partly under the nail fold and the *cuticle*.

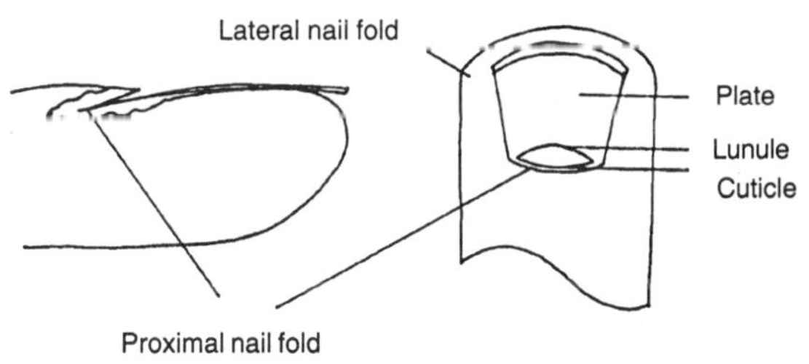

Fig. 20. Structure of the nail.

Initially the cells of the nail are soft, but as they appear from under the cuticle, they harden to appear as the nail-plate. The nail-plate is made up of layers of dead keratin cells, which are bound together by a natural glue of fats (phospholipids) and water. The shape of the nail is determined by your bone structure; if your fingers are long and fine, your nails will be long and relatively narrow but if your bones are wide, your nails will be flat and square-shaped.

Your nails reflect your body health

Several things that happen to your body get registered in your nails, for instance, if you have suffered recently from a severe illness, this illness interferes with the growing part of the nail, producing a ridge or a furrow in the nail. Taking into account the growth rate of the nail the doctor can tell by examining the nails, roughly when the illness took place.

Unlike the hair, nails grow continuously throughout life and are not normally shed. If at all they are shed, they are replaced at about the same rate as the normal nail. The fingernails normally grow at the rate of about 1 mm per week. So it takes, on an average, about six months for the whole nail to be replaced. The toenails grow at a slower rate. The growth of the nail also slows down with age — this is because the blood supply of the hands and feet decreases as age increases. The nail growth is also slower in winter.

Poor diet is often the cause of bad nails. Deficiency of iron causes spooning of nails — a condition called *koilonychia*. Your diet should also include proteins (meat, fish, cheese, soyabeans), vitamins and minerals like calcium, for the maintenance and growth of nails. The popular belief that eating gelatin can improve the condition of your nails, is somewhat scientific because gelatin is nothing but protein.

NAIL DAMAGE AND ITS PREVENTION

Nail damage due to household chores

Modern kitchen chemicals — detergents, washing powders and bleaches are all very powerful chemicals and can cause a number of nail problems. Further, your nails are soaked in water several times every day — when you wash dishes, clothes and floors etc. Even more damaging to the nails is the effect of incompletely drying your hands — the kitchen cloth is usually damp or missing when you have to hurriedly attend to the door bell or have to run to change the baby's diapers. Then there are other chores damaging to the nails; gardening, dialing the phone, opening tins — all these cause a variety of physical injuries to the nails. So if you do not care for them, your nails will flake and become brittle and really look awful.

How to avoid damage to your nails?

The simplest way is to use gloves. A lot of women argue that they just cannot do household chores wearing gloves; if you buy a pair of comfortable and good gloves, there is no reason why you should not be able to do most domestic chores wearing them. After all, do not surgeons perform the finest of surgeries wearing gloves! It is important that your gloves are large and comfortable; and don't wear them for more than half an hour at a time, because they themselves may then cause problems.

If you simply can't wear gloves, you could at least use a long-handled mop — this allows you to keep your hands out of water and your nails will definitely benefit. If you do get your hands wet, remember to rinse them well and dry them carefully after the work is done. Then apply ample amounts of a moisturising cream.

You must also take certain other precautions : use a pencil to operate the dial, use a tin-opener to open tins, use gardening gloves, avoid contact with strong chemicals, use moisturisers liberally.

PAMPER YOURSELF

Give yourself a manicure

Healthy, well-groomed nails make for an attractive appearance. You can reveal the natural beauty of your nails by following this step-by-step guide to a do-it-yourself manicure. It takes less than twenty minutes, costs you almost nothing and will leave your nails looking strikingly beautiful.

What you would need are (Fig. 21A): *(a)* a bowl of water with half a tablespoon of shampoo added, *(b)* hand cream, *(c)* enamel remover, *(d)* emery board, *(e)* nail clippers, *(f)* a pair of sharp curved scissors or cuticle trimmer, *(g)* orange stick, *(h)* a soft sponge, *(i)* cotton wool, and *(j)* hand towel.

1. After removing the old enamel, soak the hands in the bowl of soapy water for 5 minutes. Clean your nails using a soft sponge. Then dry your hands and nails thoroughly.
2. Clip the nails to the desired length. Don't clip them too far down the side of the nail.
3. Using an emery board, smooth out the edge of each nail to a good shape. File the nails only in one direction from the side to the centre (Fig. 21 B), because if you file the nails with a sawing to-and-fro movement, the edges are abraded and are likely to chip off. Use the rough side of the emery board to shape the nails and the fine side to smoothen the rough edges. Avoid filing far down into the corners of the nails, as the tips are less likely to break if they are supported by straight sides extending about an eighth of an inch beyond the flesh of the finger (Fig. 21C).
4. Bevel the edges of the nails by holding the board at an angle of 45° to the nail tip and working the fine edge in an upward direction from under the free edge (Fig. 21D). Bevelling reduces the chance of the nails breaking.
5. Check the symmetry of the shape of the nails by looking at them with the palm facing you (Fig. 21E).

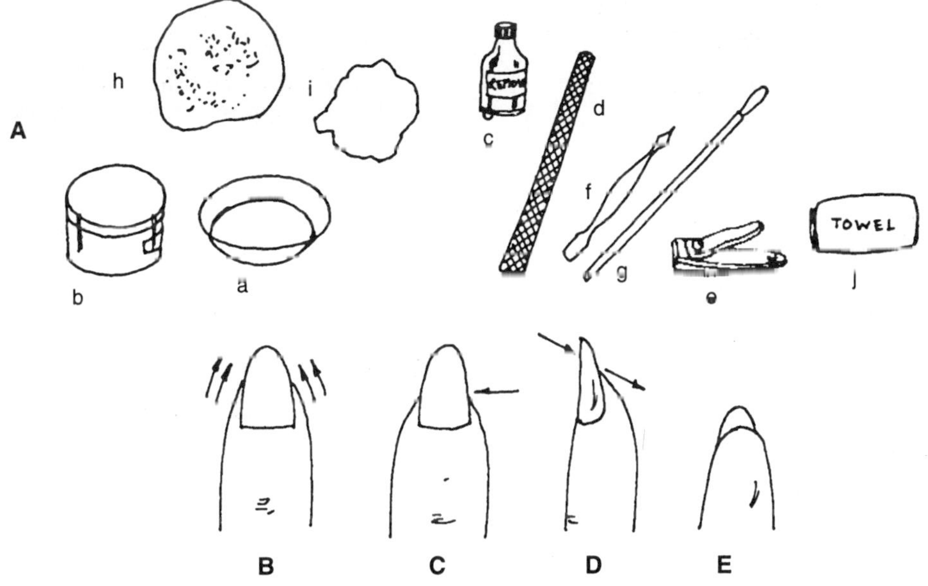

Fig. 21. Give yourself a manicure.

6. Soften the cuticles with soapy water. Gently release the cuticle of each nail using an orange stick. Avoid manipulating the cuticle with sharp instruments because once the cuticle is injured, your nails are in trouble.
7. Using a small pair of sharp clippers, trim off any ragged and rough skin that is present around the nails (Fig. 21F).
8. Using an orange stick padded with cotton wool, gently clean under each nail to remove any remaining dirt (Fig. 21G).
9. Apply cream to the cuticles. Massage the fingers using plenty of hand cream, using rotating movements towards the finger tips. Rub in the excess cream on to the rest of the hand.

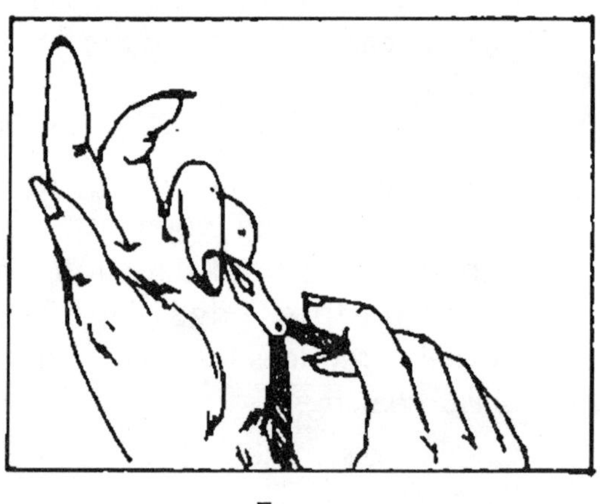

F

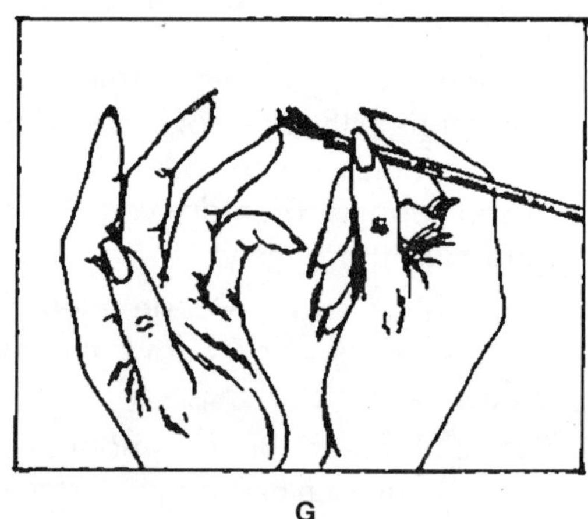

G

Fig. 21. Give yourself a manicure.

Don't ignore your toenails

Many of us look after our fingernails very diligently but totally ignore the toenails. Remember your toenails do exist and are longing to be looked after too!

Before you begin, get the following together (Fig. 22A): *(a)* a tub of soap water, *(b)* nail-file, *(c)* nail-clippers, *(d)* an orange stick, *(e)* cotton wool, *(f)* massage cream, and pumice stone.

Sit comfortably, placing your feet on a stool.

1. Clip your toenails straight and keep them short (Fig. 22B). Toenails don't look too good when kept long.
2. Smooth down any rough edges using a triple cut steel file. File in the same direction (Fig. 22C). Never shape the toenails as this will encourage development of ingrowing toenails.
3. With a pumice stone smooth away any rough skin, after soaking the feet for about 15 minutes in a basin of soapy water.
4. Place cream on each toenail and work it into the cuticles with an orange stick, easing the skin away from the nails (Fig. 22D); don't use any sharp instruments and don't use force.

5. Rub a generous amount of cream all over the feet in smooth upward strokes.
6. Your toenails are now ready to be painted.

Those were the 6 steps to glamorous toes.

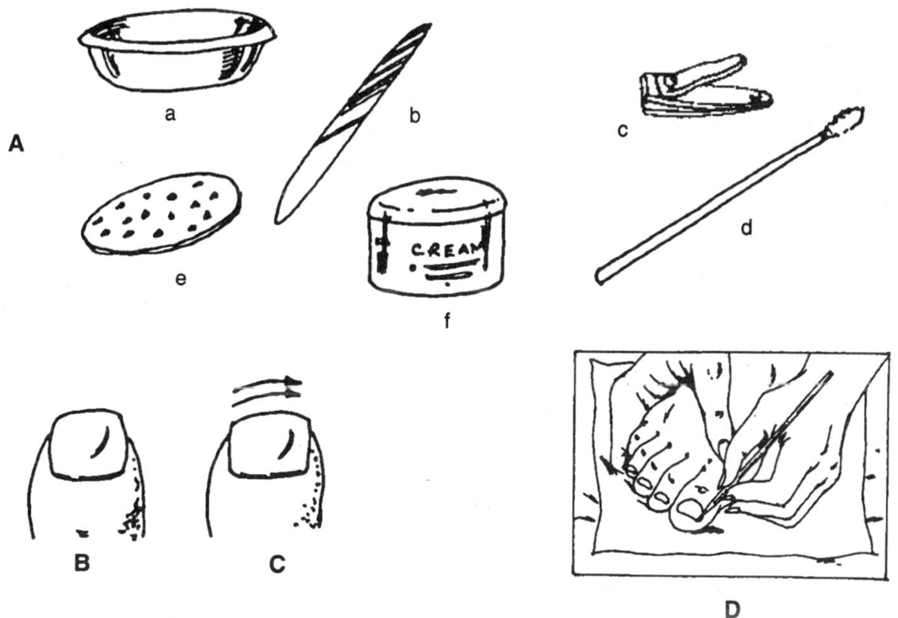

Fig. 22. Give yourself a pedicure.

COSMETICS FOR NAILS

Cosmetics for nails include not only nail polishes, but also preformed nails, sculptured nails, and nail-mending cos-metics. Most women routinely use only nail polishes but it is always worthwhile to know about the other specialised cosmetics available for your service, in case you ever need to use them.

Nail lacquers

This is the term used for all nail covering cosmetics; nail enamels, top-coats, and base-coats.

Base-coats are used to improve the adhesion of the nail enamel to the nail. They do not contain colouring agents. They may contain additives like gelatin which are thought to improve the quality of the nails.

Top-coats improve the depth and lustre of the enamel and also increase the resistance of the enamel to chipping and abrasion. They are also colourless but may contain sunscreens to protect the nails from sunlight.

All *nail enamels* contain cellulose nitrate. Different pigments are added and today there is such an enormous range of colours and finish available in nail enamels.

Nail polish is not bad for your nails

People often say that wearing nail polish all the time is harmful because the nails cannot 'breathe'. This notion is totally absurd, because the part of the nail which is painted is dead and anyway does not breathe. On the contrary, if your nails are weak, enamel can actually give it some degree of protection by guarding against breakage as it binds the fragile and flaking nails. Polishes which contain nylon or acrylic also strengthen the nail by forming a thick coat. For nails which break or flake easily, a colourless polish or a base or top-coat can be used with advantage because you can keep touching it up without having to remove the original coat.

The main problem with the use of nail polish is that associated with their use, the use of polish remover. These are very drying because they remove the natural fats from the nails. So the frequent use of removers can cause nail problems and must be avoided.

In some people nail polishes do cause allergic reactions. Rashes can appear on any part of the body which comes in contact with the nails — eyelids, face, and sides of the neck. The nails themselves are not affected though the adjoining skin may be involved.

A minor problem with the use of nail enamel is the staining of the nails — this occurs more frequently with certain enamel colours like pink and magenta. The staining gradually fades if you stop using the nail enamel.

Cosmetics to disguise nail defects

If your nails are deformed, the first thing to do is to visit your dermatologist — a number of nail problems are easily and cheaply treated. Most nail problems are temporary and improve as the new nail appears and only a very few are permanent.

The appearance of your nails can also be improved considerably by the use of cosmetics — for instance, ordinary nail enamel can camouflage a number of nail defects. A broken or split nail can be mended using what are called nail-mending fluids. To do this, a piece of thin tissue is placed over the crack or break in the nail. The nail mending fluid is then applied. When the product dries and sets, the nail can be painted with the nail enamel.

Artificial nails

There are two types of artificial nails available — preformed plastic nails and sculptured nails. You can form nails of the desired length using them. Preformed plastic nails are trimmed to the wanted shape and length and affixed with a special adhesive supplied with the kit. Some natural nail plate surface must be present to allow the adhesion of the plastic nails. So if your nails are totally lost, then plastic nails cannot be used.

Since it is time consuming to apply them to all the 10 nails, preformed nails are generally useful if only 1-2 nails are deformed. Moreover, these should not be worn continuously for more than a couple of days, as they themselves are known to cause damage to the existing nails.

Sculptured artificial nails are also called finger nail elongators. Here also some natural nail must be present. The natural nail is painted with the acrylic compound which hardens to produce the prosthetic nail. This prosthesis is filed and manicured to the desired shape. As the nail plate grows out, further application of the acrylic can be made to maintain a regular contour. These artificial nails can themselves also cause several problems and so are of little practical use.

COMMON NAIL PROBLEMS

White patches in the nails are not caused by calcium deficiency

There are a number of causes for the appearance of white patches in the nails, but calcium deficiency is not one of them. Immature nail cells are soft and reflect light and so appear white. As the nail grows these cells normally harden forming the normal transparent nail. Damage to the growing portion of the nail, for instance, due to any kind of physical injury, can interfere with the hardening of the cells of the nail. As a result, some cells retain their ability to reflect light and appear on the surface either as white spots or as white streaks.

The normal free edge of the nail also appears white because it is not attached to the nail bed and reflects light. Similarly, any nail problem which causes separation of the nail plate from the nail bed can cause whitish streaks on the nail. A common cause of such white patches is fungal infection of the nail — this problem must be shown to the doctor for treatment.

What causes brittle nails? How can you avoid this problem?

Brittle nails and flaking of nails are very common due to excessive dryness of the nail plate. As mentioned earlier, the nail plate is made up of dead keratin cells held together by a natural glue of fats and water. Any loss of fats and water causes the cells to separate and results in flaking and brittleness of the nails.

Many of our domestic chores (washing, mopping and scrubbing) remove the natural fats from the nails resulting in brittle nails. To avoid this, do wear rubber gloves for household chores — this really does help!

Nail polish removers also have a dehydrating effect. If your nails are brittle you must definitely avoid removing your nail polish too frequently. Instead, if possible, you should paint a new colour over the old one or skilfully patch up the chipped enamel. Another alternative is to use a colourless polish or a base-coat or a top-coat, because then you can keep touching it up quite happily, without having to use the remover very frequently.

If you must use enamel remover, always rinse off the excess after removing the polish. Avoid using acetone (which is cheaper) because it has a much stronger drying effect than the purpose-made formulae, which are mixtures of acetone and esters with a little oil added to decrease the drying effect.

Regular massage around the nail-base with cream can have a good effect on brittle nails. This stimulates circulation around the nail as well as protects the skin from excessive dryness. However, the more expensive creams with exotic additives like gelatin cannot do much more than ordinary creams, except that they make a large dent in your pocket.

Hangnails

Hangnails are tears in the skin of the nailfolds and the cuticle. The cuticle and the nailfolds have a tendency to stick to the nail-plate as it grows forward; the stretched cuticle may eventually tear. Sometimes the skin of the nailfolds also cracks, particularly if it is dry. Nervous habits such as biting nails, chewing nails and picking the cuticle, all encourage the development of hangnails.

To avoid hangnails, keep the cuticles soft by massaging in creams and regularly loosening it from the nail-plate. When you are loosening the cuticle from the nail-plate, be gentle. Existing hangnails are best clipped off; avoid pulling off the slivers as this can be very painful and can even cause infection of the nailfolds.

What causes paronychia?

Paronychia is inflammation of the nail-folds, which become swollen, painful and red. In severe types pus may ooze from the nailfolds. Too frequent and prolonged immersion of the hands in water is the primary cause of paronychia. Once the damage to the skin has occurred, infection by fungus and bacteria may supervene. It is commonly seen in housewives, kitchen helpers, bakers and dishwashers.

Paronychia can easily be prevented, if you keep your hands as dry as possible, if you dry wet hands carefully, if you use rubber gloves (especially if your hands have to be in contact with water for long periods of time), and if you handle the nail-cuticle carefully. Once the problem has set in, seek expert help — you might require medication with antibiotics and anti-fungal agents.

Prevent in-growing toenails

If the toenail is not cut properly, it penetrates into the nail-fold as it grows, causing redness, swelling and pain. Those of you who have had this problem would know that not only it is very painful, but physically incapacitating too.

The best way to avoid an in-growing toe nail is to ensure that your toenails are cut properly. There are three cardinal rules to follow when you are trimming your toenails:

- Don't cut them too short.
- Don't ever cut down the side of the nail.
- Always follow the shape of the toe.

Ideally the free edge of the nail should rest on the tip of the toe so that it is not possible for it to pierce the adjoining skin as it grows. If you cut the nail too short, it is easy to push the nail fold around it and encourage problems. Also if you cut down the side of the nail-plate, as the nail grows its sharp free edge penetrates the adjacent skin causing considerable pain.

Once the pain has started, try to push the nail-fold away from the sharp edge of the skin. Do this regularly, till the nail has grown out. If the nail fold is swollen and there is pus discharge, it is best to call on your dermatologist. The doctor would initially try to manoeuvre the nail edge out; if this fails, then the nail might have to be cut and removed.

Fungal infections of the nail

Fungus can infect any part of the body. Infection of the nails by fungus is called *onychomycosis*. The nails are thickened, broken and discoloured. Fungal infection can easily be treated – *griseofulvin* is an effective therapy but needs to be given for about 6 months (for finger nails) to 9 months (in case of toe nails). *Terbenafine* is a newer antifungal, which needs to be used only for 2-3 months, but it is definitely more expensive.

●●●

7. Teeth and Mouth Care

STRUCTURE AND DEVELOPMENT

Structure

Human beings develop 2 sets of teeth in their lifetime; the primary dentition (baby teeth or milk teeth) and the permanent dentition which replaces the primary set during childhood. There are 20 teeth in the primary set and 32 teeth in the permanent set. In the adult, in each quadrant from the midline, there are 2 incisors, 1 canine, 1 premolar and 3 molars.

Each tooth is composed of a *crown* and one or more *roots* (Fig. 23). The crown is the portion of the tooth which projects into the oral cavity. Its shape varies from tooth to tooth, depending on its function. The roots of the teeth are the portions which are contained within the bony socket. The roots are attached to the bony socket by means of the *periodontal fibres* which hold the teeth firmly in place.

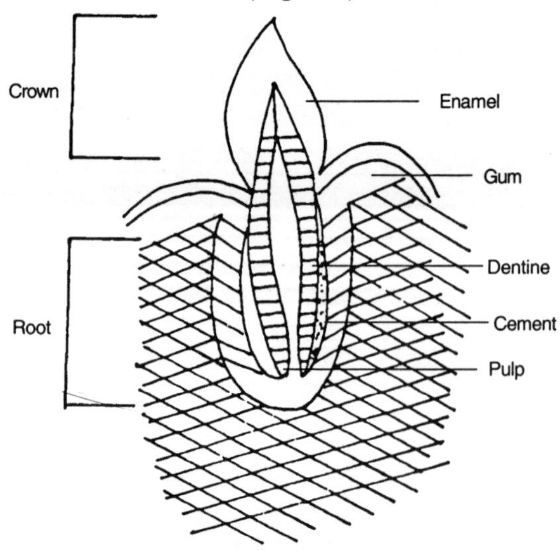

Fig. 23. Structure of the tooth.

The bulk of the tooth is made up of *dentine*, but the crown is covered by a layer of *enamel*. Enamel is the hardest structure in the body. The roots are covered by a thin layer of *cement*. The tooth has a hollow centre which contains the *pulp*. This holds the blood vessels and nerves of the teeth.

Development

The ages at which the individual teeth erupt are very variable, even the order in which they erupt varies. The primary teeth start to form before birth. On an average, they begin to erupt at 6 months and by the age of 3, the milk dentition is fully established. When newly erupted, these teeth are arranged in close contact with each other, but by the age of 6 years, when the permanent teeth start to replace them, they are well spaced, because of the growth of the jaws.

At the age of six-and-a-half years, the first permanent molars erupt. Shortly afterwards, the primary teeth begin to shed and are replaced by their permanent successors. Between the ages of 7 and 12 years all other primary teeth are replaced. Finally between the ages of 17 and 21 years the third molars erupt. When they first appear in the mouth, the permanent teeth are also crowded together, but with the continuing growth of the jaws, they straighten themselves out, although in many cases, some degree of crowding remains.

Ideally, the jaws come together with the upper incisors closing over the lower ones by an overbite of approximately 2 mm. They also project in front of them by an overjet of about 2 mm (Fig. 24). The upper canines occlude behind the lower. Each upper tooth except the last, occludes with 2 lower teeth.

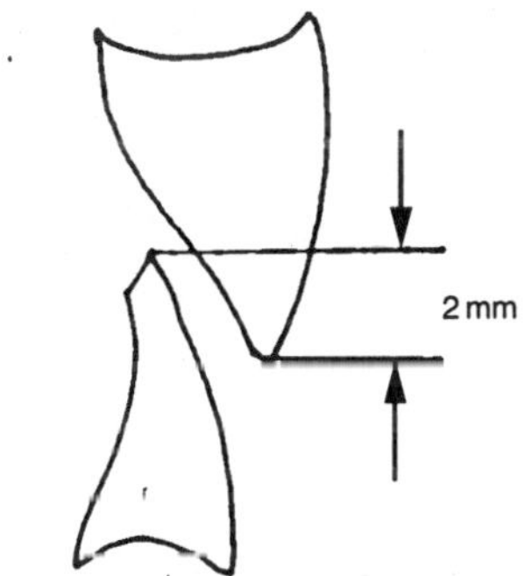

Fig. 24. How the jaw closes — a side view of the front teeth.

REGULAR CLEANING OF TEETH

The toothbrush

In the past, an inordinate amount of time has been devoted to discussing toothbrush design; so there are a multitude of different shapes and sizes of toothbrushes available. It is, however, best to use a simply designed or slightly angulated toothbrush. A brush with a head approximately 2.5 cm in length is ideal for use in an average adult. Nylon bristles are superior to natural bristles because they are more hygienic and are easier to maintain. Medium textured brushes are the best because they cause very little injury to the gums.

How often should one replace the brush? Generally, the bristles of the medium toothbrush splay in about 4-6 weeks. This is when the brush needs to be replaced.

How frequently should you brush your teeth?

Ideally teeth should be brushed immediately after each meal. Brushing before going to bed is most important because during sleep the flow of saliva is reduced and any food that is retained in the mouth during the night causes the most of the damage.

Technique of brushing

The object of brushing the teeth is to remove all '*plaque*' from every accessible teeth surface without causing damage to the teeth and the gums. A methodical approach should be adopted so that all the surfaces of all the teeth are brushed.

The brush is laid against the gums and the teeth, so that its bristles point towards the root (Fig. 25A). The head of the brush is then rotated, pulling its bristles down along the gums on to the teeth in the direction of the tooth eruption (Fig. 25B and C). The brushing technique should be used systematically first on the upper jaw, then on the lower jaw. Begin on the outer aspects of the last teeth on one side, and work around via the front teeth to the last teeth on the other side. The process is then repeated for the inner surface of the teeth. Finally, the biting surface is cleaned by moving the brush back and forth. Each area should be brushed at least ten times, ensuring maximum cleanliness of the teeth and maximum stimulation of the gums.

What is the use of dental floss?

The toothbrush cannot adequately clean in between the teeth. Dental floss is the most efficient method to clean this area. Waxed and unwaxed floss is available. The floss is wrapped around two fingers and gently pulled backwards and forwards between the teeth, taking care to avoid damage to the gums. It is best to learn this technique from your dentist.

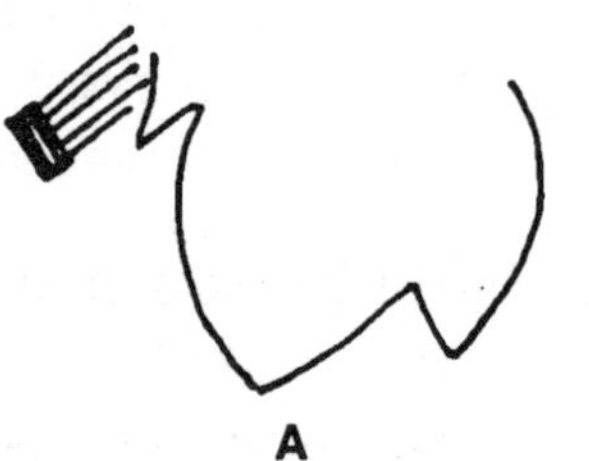

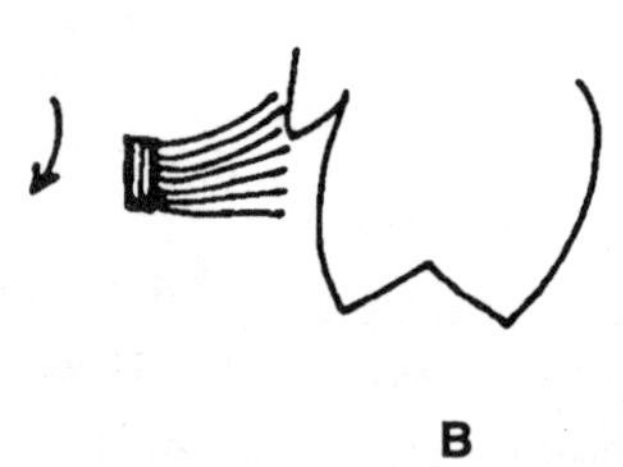

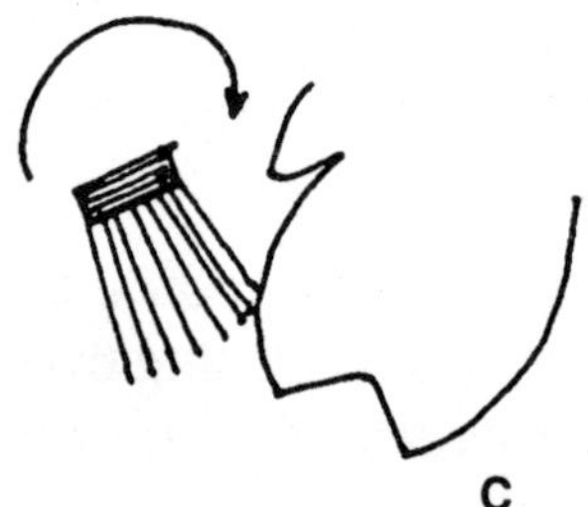

Fig. 25. The brushing technique.

Which toothpaste to use?

Toothpastes are supplementary to the brush – they aid in the cleaning and polishing of accessible surfaces of the teeth. The main constituents of toothpastes are mild abrasives, soaps, detergents, colouring agents and flavouring agents. Additional substances such as ammonium salts, chlorophyll, fluorides and cloves have been used with varying degrees of success. The value of fluorinated toothpastes in preventing caries is now definite.

If a commercial paste is not available, salt and bicarb of soda are very cheap and effective substitutes. It is, however, a bad practice to rub lime juice on the teeth as it can damage the teeth.

The dentist and oral hygiene

For good teeth, regular visit to the dentist is necessary. His role is to ensure the complete elimination of decay and stagnation. This is done by scaling, polishing and filling the teeth and carrying out corrective techniques as and when necessary. This ensures that there is no region in the mouth where food can lodge and cause problems. Further, he would advise you on the techniques of oral hygiene. A visit once in 6 months is usually adequate.

DIET AND YOUR TEETH

Fluorides

A very important line of defence lies in improving the structure of teeth by ensuring that a balanced diet is taken during tooth formation. Thus, adequate intake of calcium, phosphorus, fluoride and vitamins A, C & D are essential. Most of these are present in adequate amounts in the normal balanced diet. Only fluoride tends to be deficient and needs to be supplemented. The additional fluoride is usually provided by artificially fluoridating the drinking water (if it contains less than 1 part of fluoride per million parts of water). Teeth containing fluoride are definitely more resistant to decay.

Carbohydrates

There is a definite relationship between caries (tooth decay) and the intake of carbohydrates, especially the intake of refined carbohydrates. By refined carbohydrates we mean flour, sugar and other carbohydrates which have been treated in order to make them whiter, less fibrous and tastier. Refined carbohydrates become sticky quickly and cling to the teeth for long periods. They are then easily broken down to acids by the bacteria in the mouth — these acids are primarily responsible for tooth decay. Furthermore, it is the frequent consumption of sweet, sticky snacks which causes the worst damage. This is because the more frequently sugar is consumed, the greater is the period during which the acid is available to attack the teeth.

In view of the relationship between caries and refined carbohydrates, their intake should be strictly controlled. Ideally, they should be completely eliminated. This is a rather difficult proposition because a large number of foods contain 'invisible' sugars and it is often difficult to eliminate these foods from our diet; for instance, ketchups contain about 30% sugar, and wafer biscuits about 45%. The best would be to stick to natural unprocessed foods – meat, fish, eggs, fats, cereals, vegetables, fruits and cheese. Vegetables contain 2-3% sugar which is safe and fresh fruits rarely contain more than 12%. The only natural food which has a high sugar content is honey (76%) and this is best avoided. The sugar substitutes like saccharin also do not cause caries.

Other foodstuffs

Frequent consumption of acidic foodstuffs (like habitual drinking of carbonated drinks and excessive consumption of some fruit juices) is associated with erosions of the teeth. The best way to prevent tooth decay due to fruit juices and soft drinks is to drink them using straw. It has been suggested that fried foods coat the teeth and protect them from contact with dangerous acids and hence prevent tooth decay. It has also been suggested that one should end meals with fibrous foods such as carrots and other salads. This is because it is thought that fibrous foods might have a mild cleansing action as they remove food debris from the teeth. In addition, they might stimulate the periodontal tissues. Moreover, It Is definitely better to end a meal with fibrous foods rather than with sweets and desserts which are definitely harmful.

DENTAL CARIES

What causes dental caries?

Dental caries is nothing but tooth decay. It is the disease of the hard parts of the teeth, leading to their disintegration. Bacteria are normally present in the mouth. Some of these such as *lactobacilli* act on the carbohydrates (especially refined carbohydrates) to break them down first to simple sugars and then to acids. These acids diffuse around the teeth and literally dissolve the mineral resulting in a hole. Holes occur most frequently in the recessed areas of the teeth – where two adjoining teeth meet, in the natural fissures on the chewing surfaces of the back teeth, and on the surface of the teeth next to the gum. These are the areas from where the brush cannot remove the *plaque* of bacteria.

Can you stop decay by brushing your teeth?

The simple answer is 'no'. The film of bacteria known as the *plaque* reforms so quickly after brushing, that you would have to clean the teeth perfectly, including 'the hidden areas', every hour or so to be 'plaque free'. And this is clearly impractical.

Moreover, the bacterial *plaque* is only one of the factors in the causation of caries. The structure of the tooth itself influences the occurrence of caries. Tooth decay occurs most readily in stagnation areas, for instance, caries is common in the pits and fissures of teeth. These areas cannot be reached by even the fine bristles of the toothbrush and the *plaque* there remains undisturbed despite frequent brushing. Abnormally placed teeth also prevent adequate natural and artificial cleansing and therefore lead to stagnation.

The only successful way to stop decay is to cut down on the frequency of eating sugar. This is not as easy as it sounds, because sugar is often present 'invisibly' in many foods. Adequate brushing alone will also not eliminate decay, but it does stop the plaque film from building up to a great thickness and so cuts down on the acid production.

Your dentist's role in management of caries

Since caries is usually symptomless unless it has become deep and badly infected, regular visits to the dentist would assist in the early detection of caries. At this stage, caries is totally reversible just by topical application of fluorides. Further, the dentist could seal the deep fissures, which are inaccessible to cleaning and so very prone to decay. In case teeth are malpositioned, the dentist could straighten them out by orthodontic treatment. This would help you to maintain a better oral hygiene. If caries is well established, the dentist would be required to fill the cavities or give more specialised treatments like root canal treatment.

Does fluoride really help to prevent tooth decay?

Yes it definitely does. There is clear evidence that people who live in an area which has an optimal level of fluoride in the water, suffer much less from tooth decay. Fluoride makes the tooth less soluble and more resistant to acid attack. Ideally, the teeth should be exposed to fluoride during tooth formation and this is best achieved by drinking fluoridated water. When taken by mouth, during the period of tooth formation, fluoride is incorporated into the structure of the teeth.

Though the greatest beneficial effects of fluoride on teeth are seen if it is taken systemically, topical fluorides also help in building strong teeth. Topical fluorides can reverse the early caries and arrest the more established caries. Also even when systemic fluorides have been used on a regular basis, topical fluorides provide an additional protection.

The main ways of applying fluorides are: *(a)* topical solutions like *sodium* and *stannous fluorides* used by dentists; *(b)* mouth washes which are used weekly (0.20% *sodium fluoride*) or daily (0.05% *sodium fluoride*); and *(c)* toothpastes which are used daily.

Eighty to ninety per cent of the toothpastes in the market today contain fluoride. Teeth have already begun to benefit dramatically from the use of these pastes as there has been an 'upto 30 per cent' reduction in the incidence of caries in the people using these toothpastes.

GUM INFLAMMATION (PYORRHOEA)

Symptoms

Inflammation of gums (pyorrhoea) is one of the commonest diseases in the world. Though initially the disease is superficial involving just the gums, it can progressively extend to involve the deeper tissues, i.e. the periodontal tissues which hold the teeth to the bones.

The biggest problem with gum inflammation is that it usually produces very few symptoms — most people suffering from this problem are totally unaware of it. The patient may, sometimes notice bleeding of gums especially while brushing the teeth. *Halitosis* or bad breath is most commonly caused by chronic inflammation of the gums. However, unless it is particularly severe, the patients tend to be unaware of it, although others may find it all too obvious.

The gums of those having this problem appear spongy and red, and the gum margin recedes away from the teeth enamel. The underlying bone is then destroyed and with advancing bone destruction, the teeth lose their support and loosen. Most patients seek advice at this stage, when considerable damage has already been done.

How can pyorrhoeas be prevented?

The primary cause of pyorrhoea is the 'bacterial *plaque*', the toxic materials which cause inflammation of the gum and the surrounding structures. So, the importance of oral hygiene cannot be over-emphasised; the quality of care is far more important than the frequency. Frequent toothbrushing is of little value in preventing gum inflammation if it is not accompanied by some form of interdental cleaning. This means that pyorrhoea is more likely to be prevented by a thorough removal of the plaque from every tooth surface at least once everyday, rather than by a less efficient, but more frequent brushing of teeth.

Malpositioned and crowded teeth make good oral hygiene more difficult to maintain — so in case the teeth are malpositioned and crowded, appropriate treatment needs to be taken. Some individuals allow their lips to part slightly when they are relaxing; these people develop inflammation of those parts of the gum exposed by the parted lips. This is because drying up of saliva results in the accumulation of the plaque. Smokers in general have a poorer oral hygiene as compared to non-smokers. It is not surprising therefore that they have more severe pyorrhoea. Forceful closure of teeth as seen in nail biters and teeth grinders also tends to worsen the state of inflammation.

Treatment

The most important aspect of this disease is prevention by good oral hygiene. Adequate cleaning of the mouth is absolutely necessary. The dentist helps by scaling and polishing the teeth. If the teeth are malpositioned, the dentist would correct the position of the teeth. If the problem has become very severe then the dentist might have to resort to surgery.

TOOTH STAINS

What are the causes of stained teeth?

Not every one of us has sparkling white teeth. This is because the teeth get discoloured with stains. These stains are most frequently due to external agents, though occasionally stains can be deposited within the structure of teeth. Extrinsic stains occur most frequently in the presence of roughened enamel, irregular teeth, decreased mastication, and poor oral hygiene.

Tobacco stains are the commonest stains seen and are a result of tobacco smoking. The colour varies from light brown to black. They are due to a very tenacious deposit and occur more frequently on the inner surfaces of the teeth. The severity of tobacco stain depends more upon the standard of oral hygiene than on the quantity of tobacco smoked.

A diffuse, dull, yellow staining of the tooth results from the discolouration of the bacterial *plaque* by dyes like turmeric in foodstuffs. Tartar or calculus is the third common stain. It is due to mineral salt deposits on a thick bacterial *plaque*. It causes a brownish stain and is seen both above and below the gum margin. This needs to be regularly removed by scaling.

Intrinsic stains are caused by fluorosis, tetracyclines taken during tooth formation and tooth decay.

CORRECTIVE DENTISTRY

What can be done for badly broken teeth?

Broken teeth or teeth which have decayed beyond repair can be fitted with a cap known as a crown. Crowns are made either of acrylic or of porcelain or of porcelain bonded to gold. Depending on the state of the tooth either a 'jacket crown' or a 'post crown' can be used.

If the damage is not severe or if the purpose of 'crowning' is cosmetic, the tooth can be filed into a peg on which the crown is cemented. This is a jacket crown. If, however, the tooth has snapped at the gumline, or if the decay is severe, a post crown is used.

Can the crown be made to match the rest of your teeth?

Yes. For the front teeth, acrylic or porcelain crowns are used; both come in a number of shades and can be matched almost exactly to your teeth. But since acrylic tends to turn yellowish with age, porcelain crowns are generally preferred. The crown is made to the shape of the tooth it is replacing and the inbuilt imperfections give it a natural look. If the tooth is in a vulnerable position where the crown could be broken, then the crown is made from procelain bonded to gold, because this type of crown is durable.

How durable is the crown?

The acrylic crowns tend to discolour with age, while the porcelain ones tend to retain the original colour. Porcelain is brittle and so a porcelain crown may occasionally fracture. If the tooth is in a vulnerable position, where the crown is likely to be broken, then porcelain can be strengthened by bonding it to gold.

Crowns may sometimes come off. This can be easily remedied. A crown which has come off can either be stuck back or replaced with a new one. However, the dentist may want to examine the stump, to make sure it is healthy and an X-ray may be required to see the condition of the root. If all is well, the crown can be easily fixed back.

What can be done for crooked teeth?

Overcrowded crooked teeth and gaps can be corrected by using braces which slowly and steadily move the roots in the right direction. The best time to start this corrective treatment is while the teeth are still growing and the jaw bones are soft. But it is equally important not to start the treatment too early as many of the problems would settle on their own. Dentists do not generally start these measures before the child is ten and may even delay it till later. Even adults can benefit from this type of correction. People have received successful orthodontic treatment even in the late twenties.

If the teeth are only slightly crooked, a brace may be all that is required, but if the overcrowding is serious, one or two teeth may have to be removed. Braces used for corrective dentistry are of two types. Fixed braces consist of wires attached to bands cemented on to the teeth so that the patient cannot remove them from the mouth. The second type are the removable braces which consist of wires and screws embedded in an acrylic plate which can be inserted in the mouth and taken out by the patients themselves.

An important aspect of corrective orthodontic treatment is the meticulous maintenance of oral hygiene as there is an increased incidence of caries and gum diseases in patients using braces. So, if you are using braces, look after the hygiene of your mouth rather carefully.

ORAL CANCER AND PRECANCEROUS LESIONS

Oral cancer is one of the six most common cancers in the world and constitutes 16-18% of all body cancers in India (the highest compared to anywhere in the world). It is common where betel quid chewing, bidi smoking, alcohol, and tobacco consumption is high. Other risk factors are poor oral hygiene, chronic irritation (e.g., rough teeth, denture and filling etc).

When to suspect?

- A non-healing ulcer in the mouth should be shown to the doctor.
- If your mouth feels sore, seek expert advice.
- Avoid betel/tobacco chewing.

●●●

8. Body Care

YOUR POSTURE

The correct posture

Your personality depends more than just on your face. If you really want to look good, hold your shoulders back, tighten your bottom, and straighten your back. Now look straight ahead at eye level, so that your head is evenly poised above the spine and your chin is at right angles to your neck. Keep your shoulders straight by pushing your chest up and out, to avoid a hunched back. Tuck in your tummy, because a bulging stomach is a feature of an unattractive posture. Initially you might have to make a conscious effort to maintain this posture, but later on it will come naturally to you. All this will give you a graceful carriage and make you feel fitter.

Your posture while you sit is also important. See that you sit in a suitable chair – the seat should be of such a height that the knee joint forms a right angle when the feet are resting on the floor. The back of the chair should conform to the shape of the spine and be firm enough to support the spine. Practise sitting down and rising up in one flowing movement, rather than in a series of awkward jerks; keep the top half of your body straight and lower yourself slowly into the chair. Once sitting, hold your back straight, keep your stomach in and your trunk pushed deep into the chair. Reaching upwards should also be a movement of the whole body, keeping your back straight and your weight evenly balanced on the balls of the feet. Remember to keep all movements relaxed and flowing, not jerky and stiff. The exercise schedule to follow will do much to improve your posture.

Observe your gait and improve upon it

From time to time, study your walking posture in shop windows, as you walk past them. Another way to check your gait is to imagine a straight line (or better still draw a straight line in the verandah) and walk exactly on that line. If you have a defective way of walking, your feet will not follow the line. Another way to find the fault with your gait is to walk barefoot with wet feet – check the impressions left by your feet. Practise regularly to get a straight line of walk. For good carriage while walking, practise walking with a book on your head.

WEIGHTY PROBLEMS

Problems on being overweight

An overweight person, apart from looking unattractive, may face a number of other problems too:

- Being overweight can actually be due to some internal disease, most commonly this is hormonal – diabetes, decreased activity of thyroid gland, adrenal gland problems and abnormalities of the ovaries.
- People who are overweight have an increased chance of developing skin infections, especially fungal infections in the folds.
- High blood pressure and heart attacks are more frequent in the obese.

So not only for looking good, but also for feeling and being fit, it is necessary for you to lose excess weight.

Counting calories

All the food you eat is a source of energy and can fatten you, but some foodstuffs are more fattening than others. For instance, weight for weight, fats are more fattening than both carbohydrates and proteins. Calories are a simple way to measure, how much energy and how much fattening potential your foods contain. Foodstuffs differ in their caloric content because of two reasons: firstly they contain varying amount of fats, proteins, and carbohydrates and secondly, they contain different amounts of water, an ingredient which truly has zero calories. Similarly, the energy you spend when working or exercising can be measured in calories. So the simple basis of a 'calorie control' diet would be to limit your calorie intake, and increase the utilisation of calories. Your body will then have to draw upon the fat stores to fill the energy gap and you would begin to lose weight.

To lose weight sensibly

The safest and the most effective way of slimming is to lose weight slowly. Crash diets should be avoided as they often fail. This is simply because they just cannot be sustained. Moreover, crash dieting can adversely affect your beauty, making you look haggard. An advantage of a gradual diet control is that your taste in foods can be adjusted over a reasonable period of time so that the craving for certain food items is reduced.

An average woman spends about 2,300 calories a day. If you want to reduce your weight, you should aim to eat about 1,200-1,300 calories daily. If you persistently eat about 1,000 calories less every day, your body will have to make up the shortfall, by using up about 100 grams of your body fat daily. So in about ten days you would be able to lose a kilo of your weight. On this diet you should not expect a rapid loss of weight. It may take you some time to lose the desired weight. Even though it would be slow, if you are steady in your diet control, you are sure to be a winner.

How fattening are high protein foods?

There is a popular notion that protein-rich foods are not fattening. This is absolutely a myth. Proteins actually provide the same number of calories per gram as carbohydrates and so are equally fattening. But protein-rich foods (and even fatty foods), do not leave the stomach as quickly as carbohydrates, so they tend to satisfy your appetite for longer periods of time and you do not feel hungry quickly. It is for this very reason that a serving of mutton appears to be far more filling than a bowl of cereal and sugar, even though the portions have been adjusted to give you precisely the same number of calories.

However, a slimming diet which recommends protein foods, such as eggs, yoghurt or fish rather than starchy and sugary foods is very likely to be rich in minerals and vitamins as well. And this makes real good nutritional sense too! On the other hand, refined carbohydrate foods can be easily eliminated from the diet without causing any deficiency of vitamins and minerals.

How to cut down on fats?

Since fats contain more than twice as many calories to a gram as carbohydrates and proteins, a low fat diet would seem to be a very sensible way to cut down on the calories in your daily meals. But this is only going to help you, if you make sure that the rest of your diet does not run out of control. The danger here lies in the fact that when you cut out on the fatty bit of your meals, you tend to feel hungry much sooner and if you succumb to your hunger-pangs, you might well end up eating more (snacks, sweets and other foods) before your next meal is due, and ruin your dietary schedule.

We consume a large amount of fat in our diet; actually 40% of our daily calorie intake is derived from fats. Half of this is visible as the oil we cook our food in, the ghee on our *paranthas* and the butter we spread on the breakfast bread. The other half, however, is not so obvious; the margarine present in the cakes and biscuits, the fat in boiled eggs and the cream in our morning cup of tea or coffee.

It is really not too difficult to reduce the fat content of a normal meal to about 25% – removing the cream from your morning cup of milk, banishing fried items off the menu and avoiding ghee on the chappatis. But if we try to get below this, our diet becomes almost unpalatable, because this would mean eliminating a variety of such necessary items of food as cheese, eggs and milk.

Diet for losing weight

For general calculations it is good to know the caloric values of the items of foods which are consumed routinely – these values are given in Table 3.

An effective diet for reducing weight normally contains about 1,200 calories. An example of such a diet is given below. There is a balance of carbohydrates (193 g), proteins (48 g) and fats (24 g) in this diet and it contains adequate amounts of vitamins and minerals too.

Breakfast : 1 cup tea
1 slice bread or 1 *idli* or
3 tablespoons of cooked porridge
1egg or 25g cottage cheese

Lunch : 1 cup soup
2 chappatis or 2 helpings of cooked rice
1 helping of dal
1 helping of seasonal vegetables
1 helping of curds
1 helping of fruits

Evening snack : 1 cup tea or coffee

Dinner : 2 chappatis or 2 helpings of cooked rice or
2 helpings of noodles
1 helping of meat, fish or dal
1 helping of seasonal vegetables
Plenty of green salads.

Table 3: Caloric values of common dietary items.

Items		Calories
Milk (1 glass skimmed)	:	70
Tea (1 cup + 1/2 teaspoon sugar)	:	20
Egg (1 boiled)	:	80
Cottage cheese (25 g)	:	70
Bread (1 large slice)	:	75
Chappati (1 medium-sized)	:	85
Rice (1 helping of 25 g)	:	87
Seasonal vegetables (1 helping of 125 g except tubers)	:	35
Dal (1 helping)	:	80
Fruit (1 helping 100 g except mangoes, grapes, bananas and chiku)	:	40
Curd (1 helping of 125 g)	:	75
Cold drinks (1 bottle)	:	80
Oil (1 teaspoon)	:	45
Sugar (1 teaspoon)	:	20

While on a weight-reducing diet there are certain foods you must avoid:

1. All fried foods: puris, pakoras, samosas, paranthas.
2. All sweets: honey, ice-creams, cakes, pastries, jams, chocolates, candies.
3. Dry fruits and nuts: peanuts, almonds, cashewnuts.
4. All alcoholic drinks.
5. Fruits: bananas, chiku, grapes, mangoes.

6. Vegetables: potatoes, arbi and other tubers.
7. Aerated drinks like the colas.

Foods which you can eat as much as desired without causing any problems:

1. Salads: carrots, radish, tomatoes, onions, cucumbers, lettuce.
2. Drinks: clear soups, lemon juice, jaljeera, buttermilk.

Cellulite — fact or fiction?

Fat is deposited under the skin in clusters of cells held together by a fibrous network of connective tissue. The pattern of fat storage in your body is partly controlled by the sex hormones. In men, the fat is stored in a fairly uniform manner. In women, on the other hand, fat is stored to a large extent, in one or two specific areas like the thighs and the buttocks. Some 'body care people' have termed the fat stored in these areas as *cellulite*.

Cellulite, according to these people, is a gel like substance made up of a mixture of fat, water and waste materials, all trapped as immovable lumps, just beneath the skin. The protagonists of this theory believe that when the connective tissue is "poisoned", it begins to expand abnormally, accumulating fat, water and body wastes — cellulite is thus formed.

Tension, fatigue, smoking, lack of exercise, alcohol, and drugs have been held responsible for the poisoning of connective tissue and formation of cellulite; these factors are thought to slow down the rate of elimination of waste materials from the body and these then collect in the connective tissues.

It stands to logic that if you eat more than you require, you would put on weight. The body can easily store this excess fat in the skin. When too much fat is stored, it tends to bulge out between the fibres of connective tissue. The overlying skin then begins to look and feel uneven and flabby. Doctors also agree that too many calories and too little exercise both contribute to this excessive collection of fat.

Doctors, however, do not regard cellulite formation as a special condition at all; they think that cellulite is nothing but a fancy name for excess fat. Chemical analysis has shown that cellulite is similar to ordinary fat. There is also no indication of the presence of any abnormal connective tissue or excess amount of water in the skin of people having excess amounts of the so-called cellulite.

What are anti-cellulite diets?

These diets claim to purify the body and to eliminate the so-called "poisoning agents". They basically contain the all too familiar list of low calorie foods — plenty of raw vegetables, skimmed milk, cheese, fish and lean meat. Logically, they exclude the so-called 'body polluters' like chocolates, chips, and alcohol — all having large amount of calories. So, naturally these anti-cellulite diets will help you lose weight.

Apart from their low calorie value, these anti-cellulite diets contain plenty of fluids, restrict salt intake and contain large amounts of iodine. Fluids are included because they are supposed to increase kidney activity and speed up the rate at which your body gets rid of the waste materials. Once the "poisons" are eliminated, the cellulite would follow. But this is a hypothetical explanation, because doctors do not believe that the kidney activity has anything to do with accumulation and elimination of fat.

Iodine is included to hasten up burning up of fat. Iodine is used up normally in the body by the thyroid gland to produce hormones which control the rate at which fuel is burnt. Including extra iodine in the diet is, however, unlikely to be of any use in speeding up the process of getting rid of fat, as the thyroid gland only needs a minute amount of iodine and this is generally provided by a normal balanced diet.

Are 'massage type' appliances useful?

There are several models of these gadgets available — small portable models can be bought for use at home. Saloons have the more powerful versions, which need trained staff to operate. These appliances basically consist of rubber pads, which are strapped to the body. On switching on the current, the muscles are stimulated to expand and contract about 40 times a minute. This forms a passive alternative to active exercises. Over a period of weeks, you can improve your muscle tone, thereby firming up the flabby flesh. So you tend to lose inches, but there is no loss of weight as there is no burning up of calories.

These passive exercises are actually only a poor substitute to active exercises, which have several other beneficial effects besides firming up muscles. These gadgets are of use for those of you who are heavily overweight and out of condition till such time that you can build up your stamina to undertake the optimum active exercises. And since the use of these gadgets requires very little physical effort, you can use them for long periods of time without getting tired. In addition, you can work on specific problem areas, such as poorly shaped thighs or a protuberant tummy.

What is the role of exercise in weight reduction?

Low calorie diets usually help you lose weight. But the loss of fat takes place uniformly, all over the body, but the shape of your body will actually not change. With dieting alone you may even lose weight from the unwanted places. For instance, you may lose weight from the face and this may even make you look ill. Sometimes, the fat continues to remain stubbornly in certain places.

The solution to all these problems lies in a good exercise schedule (along with your diet control); you would be able to shape the 'resistant' areas, like your hips, thighs and bottoms; it will also help you to firm up the relevant muscles. And most importantly, exercises will make you feel fit — really fit as a fiddle.

Which exercises are the most useful?

This would depend on several factors. If you want to work on specific areas of the body then you could do the exercises described in the forthcoming section. But if you want to exercise your whole body then walking, jogging, cycling and swimming are all excellent. The energy consumption of these exercises is listed in Table 4.

Is it possible to cure plump thighs with local creams or lotions?

No, not at all. But because of consumer gullibility, the cosmetic market is really well-stocked with various types of creams and lotions, all claiming to act against cellulite. These products fall into two main categories. One group contains enzymes which are thought to break down connective tissues and release the trapped toxic waste. The second group is based on seaweeds and contains plenty of vitamins and trace elements like iodine and is thought to aid in purification.

Doctors are absolutely sure that neither of these externally applied products are of any use because neither can these agents reach their targets so deep below the skin, nor are they capable of breaking down the pockets of the so-called 'toxic material' in the connective tissues. All that these cosmetics do, is to make a big, a real big, dent in your pockets.

Table 4: Calories spent during various activities.

Activities		Spent Calories/hr.
Sleeping	:	80
Driving	:	120
Standing	:	140
Domestic chores	:	180
Walking (4 km/hr)	:	210
Walking (6 km/hr)	:	300
Cycling (9 km/hr)	:	210
Cycling (21 km/hr)	:	660
Gardening	:	220
Swimming	:	300
Tennis	:	420
Running (16 km/hr)	:	900

EXERCISE YOUR BODY

Your posture routine

Here are some excellent exercises for improving your posture:

Exercise 1 **:** Thread a ruler behind your shoulders through the armholes of a sleeveless *kurta*. This will keep your shoulders well back.

Keep the ruler in place for about 15-30 minutes daily.

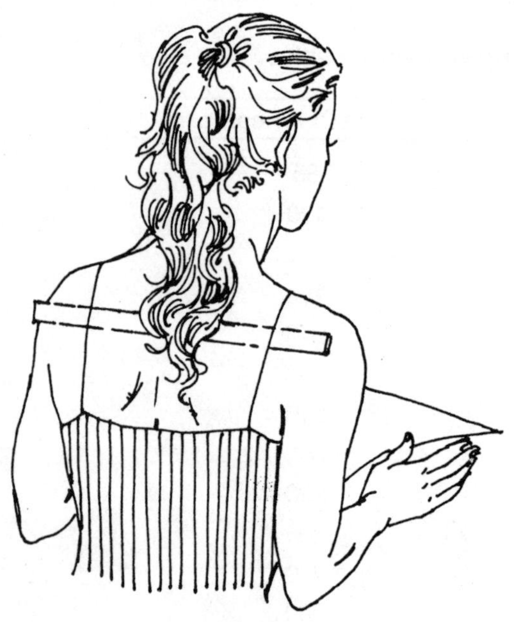

Exercise 1

Exercise 2 **:** Stand with feet slightly apart and arms held straight out on the side, at right angles to your body.

Swing both your arms backwards following a circle and then bring them back to position.

Repeat 30 times.

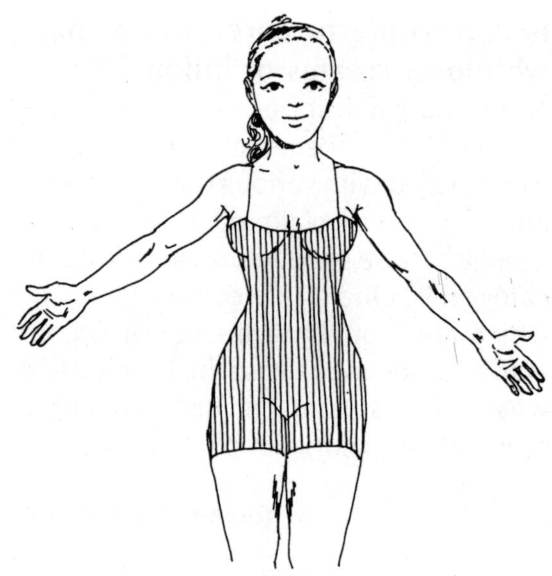

Exercise 2

Tone up your arm muscles

Exercise 3 **:** Stand with your back about one foot from the wall.

Placing your palms flat against the wall press hard against it. Hold the contraction to a count of ten.

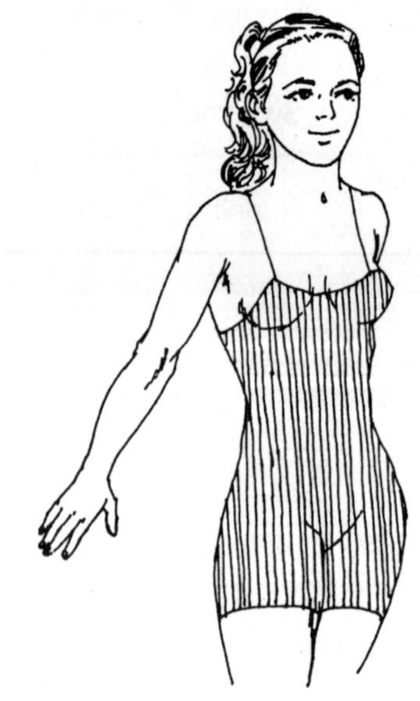

Exercise 3

Relax.

Repeat 10 times.

Repeat with your arms in front and pressing against the wall.

Repeat 10 times.

Exercises for your tired feet

***Exercise 4* :** Sit on the edge of the stool.

With legs raised, clasp your hands around your bent knees.

Rotate your feet, first outwards and then inwards, then upwards and finally downwards.

Repeat 30 times.

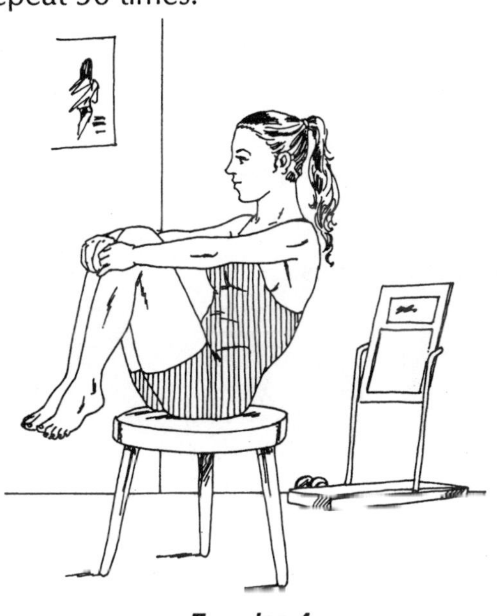

Exercise 4

***Exercise 5* :** Sit on the edge of the stool.

Place a talcum powder container on the floor. Put your right foot on it and roll it backwards and forwards from the tips of the toes to the heel.

Repeat with other foot.

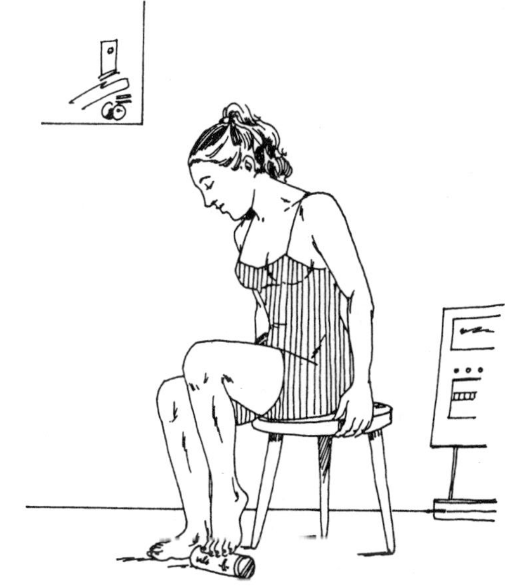

Exercise 5

Do it 10 times with each foot.

***Exercise 6* :** Sit on the floor. Bend your knees and keep back straight.

Clasp the right foot with the right hand and left foot with the left hand.

Raise left and right feet alternatively.

Repeat 10 times.

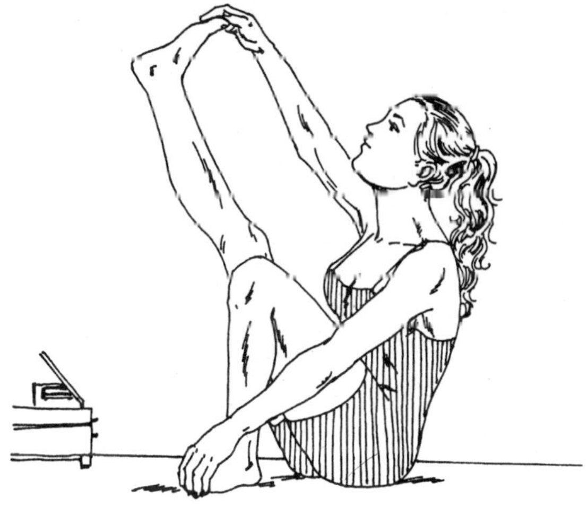

Exercise 6

Exercise 7 **:** Lie on your back with your legs raised resting against a wall.

Try to form a right angle between your legs and your body.

Stay in this position until you feel refreshed.

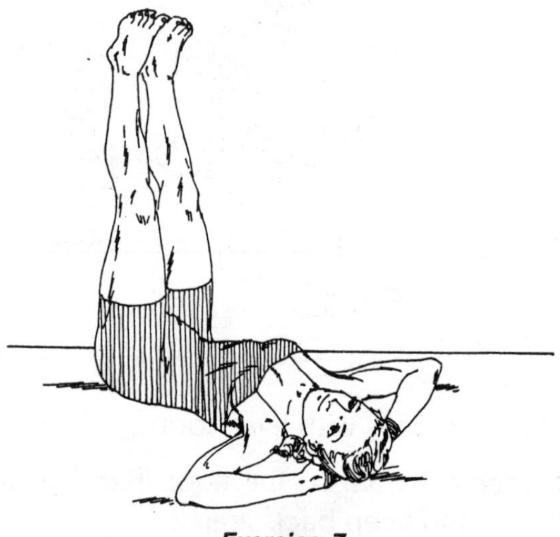

Exercise 7

Exercises for your legs

Exercise 8 **:** Stand in front of a chair, holding the handles.

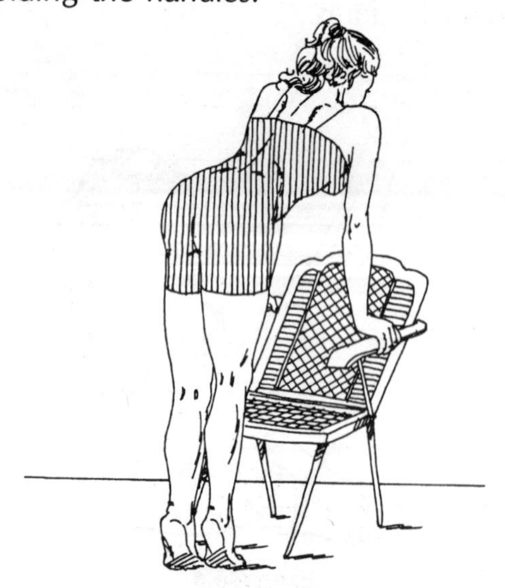

Exercise 8

Raise yourself on your toes until you are standing on tip toes.

Slowly lower the heels.

Relax.

Repeat 20 times.

Repeat with ankles far apart and toes together – 20 times.

Repeat again with ankles together and your toes far apart – 20 times.

Exercise 9 **:** Lie flat on your back on the floor.

Extend your left leg up and bend your right leg sharply from the knee in a pedalling motion; then stretch your right leg up and bend your left leg down.

Make sure that your arms remain beside your body and your hips stay firmly on the floor.

Repeat 25 times.

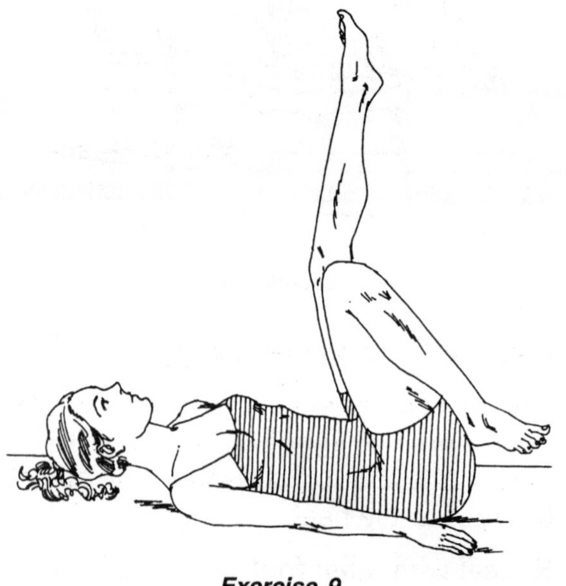

Exercise 9

Exercise 10 **:** This exercise shapes the front and back of the thighs.

Lie on the floor, on your back.

With your right leg raised straight up in the air, clasp the thigh with your hands.

Pull your thigh towards your face, while you keep your back and head on the floor.

Repeat with each leg 5 times.

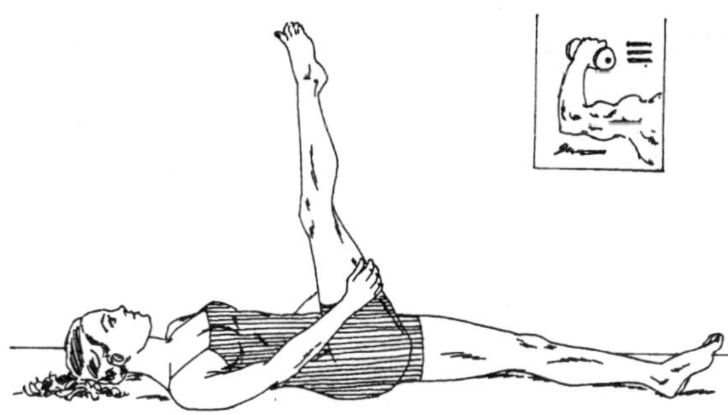

Exercise 10

Exercise 11 **:** Lie on your belly.

Elevate your right leg up straight behind you as high as possible.

Repeat with each leg 10 times.

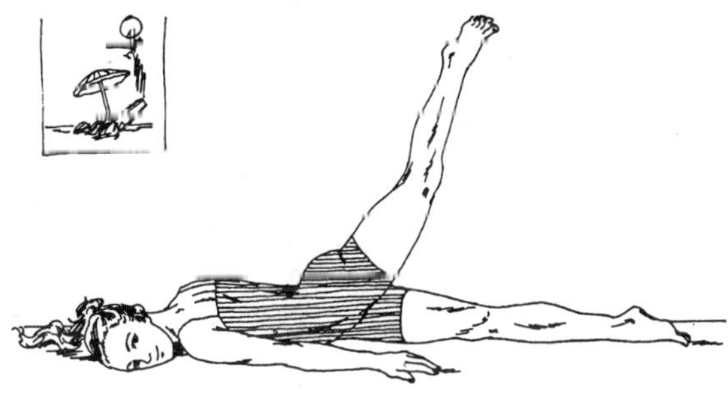

Exercise 11

Exercise 12 **:** This is to shape heavy legs.

Lying on your right side support your head on your right hand.

With your legs perfectly straight, raise your left leg to a count of five.

Hold this position for a count of five.

Slowly lower your leg to a count of five.

Repeat 10 times on each side.

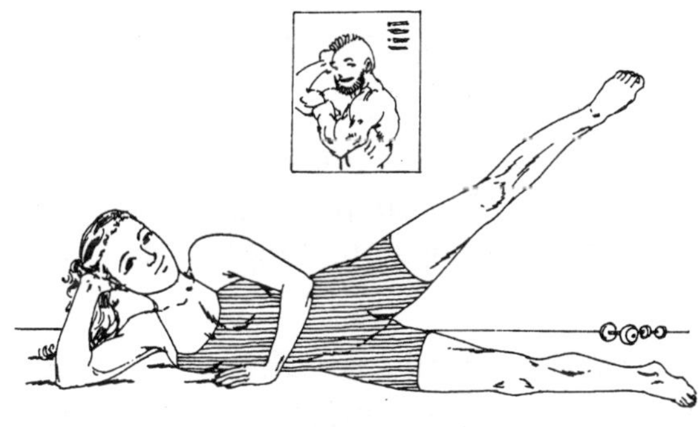

Exercise 12

Exercise 13 **:** This exercise is to streamline thighs.

Use a chairback for support and stand sideways.

Move your leg outwards in a large semicircle.

Repeat 10 times for each leg.

Exercises for your back

Exercise 14 **:** To ease tension and relax the spine, do this exercise.

Sit on the bed with your back straight and the legs apart. Rest your hands in front between your legs.

Bend your knee inwards and curl your body forward. Relax your head and arms between your legs.

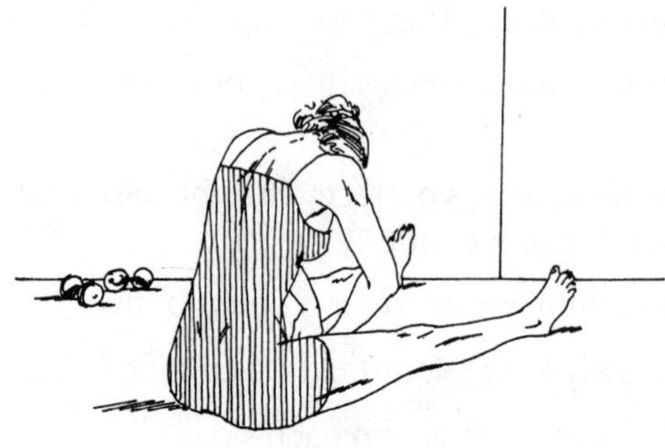

Exercise 14

Exercise 15 **:** This exercise will firm your lower back muscles.

Lie on your belly on the floor with your hands beneath you, palms pressed down and the finger tips pointing towards each other.

Raise your body off the ground, by straightening your arms and arching your spine.

Twist around to look at your feet over the right shoulder.

Repeat 5 times for each side.

Lower your body and relax to a count of 10.

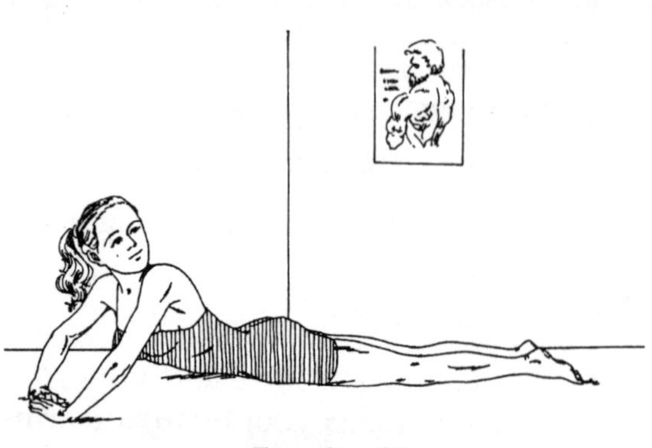

Exercise 15

Exercises for the breast

Exercise 16 **:** Lie on your tummy with the elbows bent, and fingertips facing inwards. Rest your forehead on the floor.

Slowly raise your head and body, pushing down with hands, arching your spine and bending the neck backwards.

Pull in your stomach muscles and lift your stomach off the floor.

Slowly lower upper back and shoulders to the floor to the original position.

Relax.

Repeat.

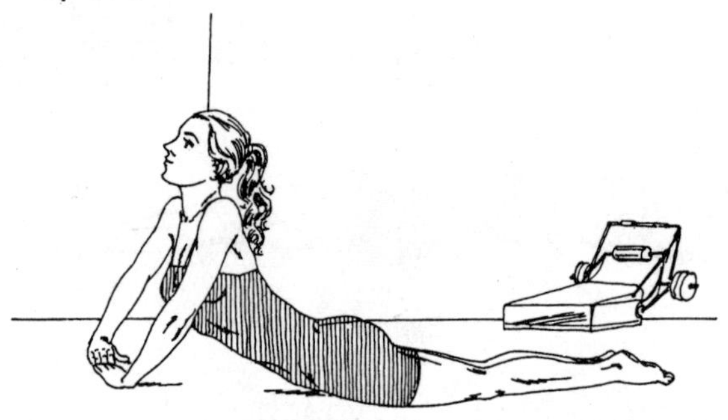

Exercise 16

Exercise 17 **:** Hold your arms straight in front of you, at shoulder level.

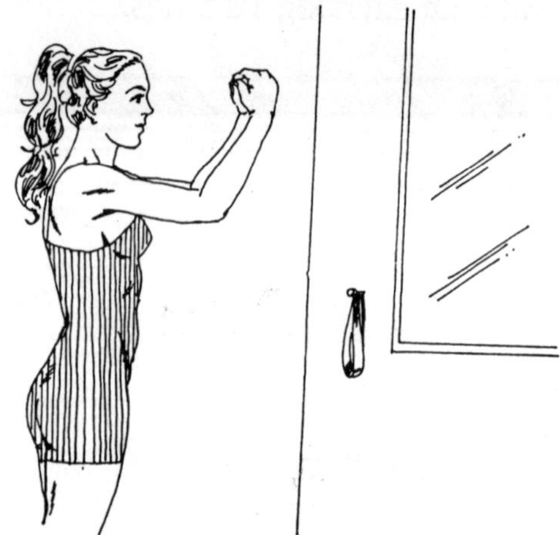

Exercise 17

Bring your hands slowly, towards your shoulders clenching your hands as though you are pulling something strenuously.

Repeat 5 times.

Exercises for a youthful bottom

Exercise 18 **:** This exercise will help to keep your buttocks firm and rounded; it also reduces fat, by reducing the effects of a sedentary life.

Sit on the floor with back straight. Point your legs straight in front of you. Fold your arms.

Walk slowly on your but-tocks.

Continue for a count of 30.

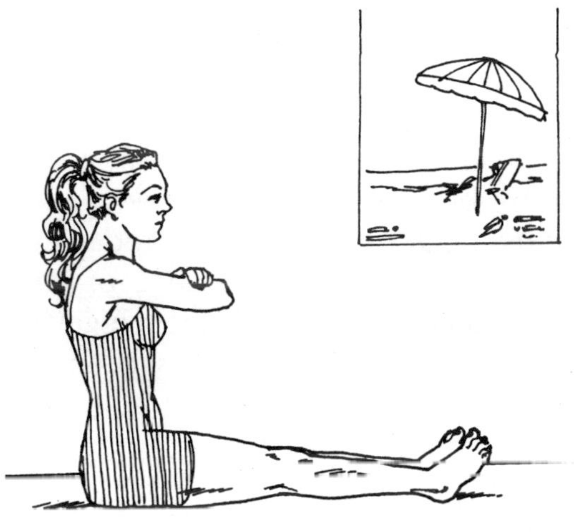

Exercise 18

Exercise while you sit

It is very important to adopt the correct posture while you sit to help keep your bottom in good shape. Too much sitting does lead to a flabby bottom. So, here is an exercise to do, while you are sitting comfortably in your chair.

Exercise 19 **:** Clasp your hands on the underside of the chair while you sit upright.

Point your legs straight out in front of you, keeping feet together, slowly raise your feet from the floor and lower them.

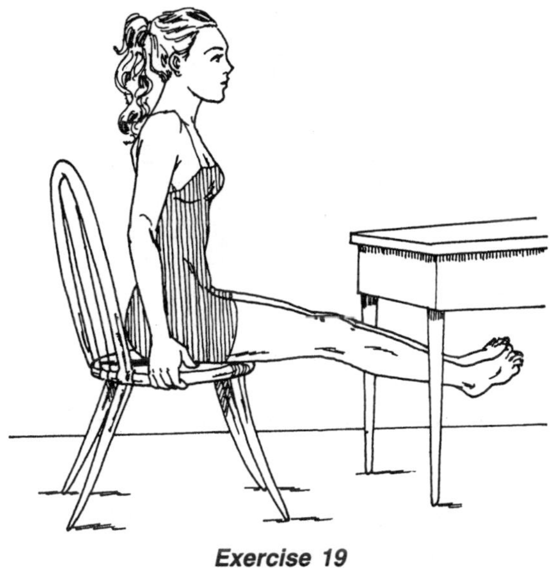

Exercise 19

Exercises for the waist and midriff

Be aware that the profile of your waist and midriff is being presented all the time – so do not slouch or stick your tummy out; instead straighten up with your shoulders back and your seat tucked in and stomach pulled in – this will keep your tummy muscles stretched, firm, flat and elegant.

Exercise 20 **:** Stand with feet apart, back straight and your hands clasped behind your head.

Twist from the waist upwards round to the right. Return to the original position and twist round to the left.

Repeat 20 times.

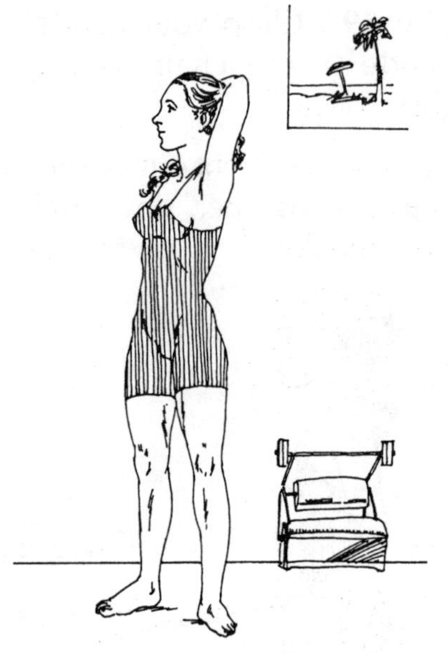

Exercise 20

Exercise 21 **:** Rest on your hands and knees.

Raise your right leg to the side keeping it straight and perpendicular to the body. Make 8 forward circles and 8 backward circles with your legs.

Repeat 5 times with each leg.

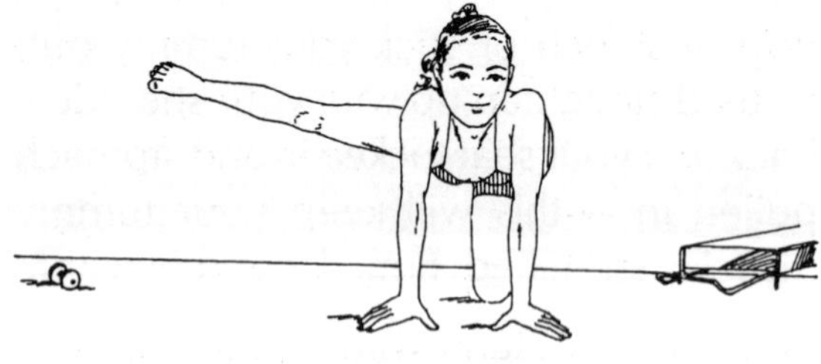

Exercise 21

Exercise 22 **:** Keep your feet apart and your arms outstretched to the side. Twisting from the waist, bend and touch your left toes with your right hand.

Return to straight position and repeat with left hand touching right foot.

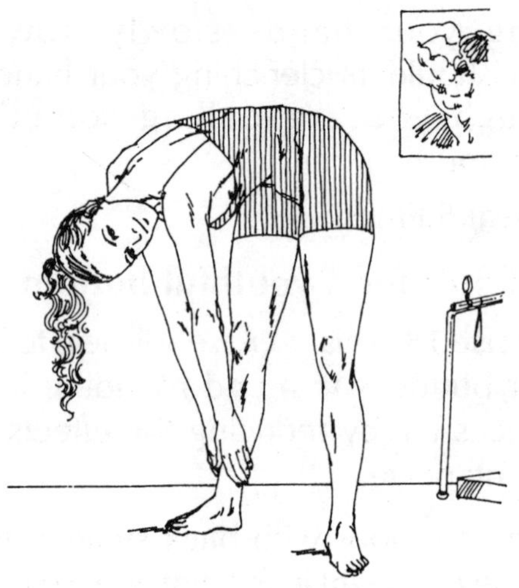

Exercise 22

Repeat 10 times.

BREAST CARE

What is your mental picture of an ideal bosom – one of small firm breasts or of sumptuous curves? Actually the essence of a beautiful and healthy bosom is firm healthy breasts – do not neglect your breasts, because regular care today can vastly improve the appearance of your breasts tomorrow. Examine them regularly for lumps and bumps as this will enable you to detect any problems early and avoid complications later.

Breasts are basically made up of cells, gland tissues, milk ducts, fibrous tissues and fat. There are no muscles in the breast tissues. The breasts would benefit greatly from a good posture, regular exercise, and reasonable support.

Supporting your breasts

Breasts have no muscles of their own and are only held up by the pectoral muscles – the muscles of the chest on which they lie. So they definitely need extra support. You can give this by wearing a good bra. Wearing a bra, which fits well, can make a great difference both to your comfort and to your contour. Most of the support that a well-fitting bra gives to the breasts should come from beneath and not the straps. You can check this by slipping off the straps to see if the bra will stay in place without them. The back-piece and the sides of a good bra should be in level with the front. If the back-piece tends to be high around the shoulder blades this could mean 2 things: that either you are hauling your breasts by the shoulder straps, or the base of the bra does not fit well. Bulging flesh at the back of the bra or at the sides and underarms means that the bra is too small.

If the bra cups are creased all over, then obviously they are too big for your breast size. To find out the correct size of the bra cup, first measure around your rib cage under your breasts. Then measure around the fullest part of your bosom at the level of the nipple. The difference between the two measurements will give you the cup size as follows:

10-12 cm	:	AA
12 14 cm	:	A
14-16 cm	:	B
16-18 cm	:	C
18-20 cm	:	D
20-22 cm	:	DD

When choosing a bra for heavy breasts, make sure it has flat well-padded undercup wiring and wide elasticized straps that give support to the centres of the breasts. Small breasts can be enhanced with the help of highly padded bras and underwiring but keep the bustline natural and do not overdo!

Will your breasts sag if you do not wear a bra?

Actually your breast will eventually sag, regardless of whether or not you have worn a bra in the past. This sagging is due to the slackening of the supporting muscles. Going braless can somewhat hasten this process, whereas a well-fitting bra will at least delay it for a little while. Sagging is more pronounced if you have large heavy breasts; if your breasts are small, you can probably get away even by not wearing a bra. Another good reason for wearing a bra is that, provided it is well-fitting, it can effectively disguise the fact that breasts may have lost some of their shape. It is also a good idea to wear a good supporting bra during vigorous exercises like running and jogging, and also during pregnancy.

What can exercise do for your breasts?

Breasts contain no muscles but only fat cells, milk ducts and glands, held together in a web of soft connective tissue. So by exercising you cannot increase your bust size. Neither will exercising directly reduce a heavy bust. This is especially true, if your breasts are large but your body weight is what it should be. If, however, you are over-weight, a weight reducing diet combined with regular exercises will help you to reduce your weight as well as your bust size.

Exercising, however, has several other advantages as well; it tones up the muscles on which the breast tissues lie. So, if your bust-line measures less than what you would like, exercises would give you a firmer and a more prominent line, making your bust appear larger. Similarly, if a heavy bust is your problem, you would lose some of the droop (which can spoil your shape) and gain a firmer contour, though there would be no loss of inches.

Apart from the exercises which we have already mentioned, swimming is a superb exercise for bust shape. It exercises the 'breast muscles' considerably against resistance of the water — this really can do wonders to your shape.

Breasts in pregnancy

During pregnancy and also during the period of breast-feeding, the breasts become larger. As the overlying skin is stretched beyond a limit, the elastic fibres in the skin tear. Red irregular marks then show up on the skin's surface. These marks are worse in some women, because the elasticity of the skin varies from person to person.

There is not very much you can do to increase the elasticity of your skin. Some people have suggested that it may be helpful to massage the skin daily. Specially formulated creams which claim to prevent stretch marks have appeared in the market. There is, however, no evidence whatsoever of the usefulness of these products. You can, however, massage the breast skin with any moisturising cream to keep it soft and supple.

The other problem the breasts face during pregnancy is sagging. In many women, breasts do return to something close to their previous shape and size, but in some the breasts become more slack and pendulous after pregnancy and breast-feeding — this again is an individual variation.

There are one or two things you can do to offset this tendency of sagging of your breasts during pregnancy: give your breasts maximum support with a good bra, wearing it day and night, and do find a few minutes everyday to exercise your supporting muscles, otherwise they will get 'lazy'. These exercises would 'tone' up your breast muscles and pep you up too!

Learn to examine your own breasts

It is important that all women know how to examine their breasts. This is important for the health of your breasts and to avoid problems later. Once you have learnt the technique, spare a few minutes every month and you would be able to pick up strange lumps and bumps at an early stage and report to your doctor.

The best time to examine your breasts is usually just after your periods, when they are at their softest. Remember, no two breasts are exactly alike — one is slightly bigger than the other and a little lower too! For breast examination, undress to the waist. Sit in front of a mirror, letting your arms hang loosely by your sides.

1. Look for a change in the size or appearance of your breasts, for any puckering or dimpling of the skin, and any change in the outline of the

breasts. Check the nipples for any discharge or bleeding.

2. For the next step, lie down on your back. Put your left hand under your head and use your right hand to examine your left breast. Use the flat of your palms and systematically examine the inner half of your breast, working your way towards the nipple. Then bring your left arm down beside, examine the outer half of the breast in the same way. Feel in the armpit too, checking carefully for any lumps. Normally too, the breasts feel rather lumpy because they are made up of milk producing glands and fat. However, this is a fairly soft and general lumpiness and both the breasts feel much the same.
3. Examine your right breast in the same way using your left hand.
4. If you find anything abnormal, consult your doctor immediately.

BODY ODOUR

Every region of the human body has a different odour; sometimes the odour is so distinctive so as to allow immediate identification of its origin. For instance, scalp and feet odours are easily recognised.

Source

There are three important factors in creating odours in your body:

1. The pattern and type of secretory glands on the skin surface.
2. The positioning of the skin itself — the armpits, for example, make it very difficult for sweat to evaporate and so produce a characteristic odour.
3. The concentration of bacteria — the skin's surface provides nutrients for the growth of bacteria. The number of bacteria are variable in different parts of the body being maximum in parts like the scalp, axilla, genital areas and the feet.

There are three types of secretory glands on the skin. Sweat glands are the most widely distributed — some two to three million such glands are present in the skin. The most important function of the sweat glands is temperature regulation. The activity of the sweat glands is controlled by the brain, depending on the temperature of the blood which is bathing the brain. The average person loses at least half a litre of sweat everyday, though this figure can rise to something like twenty litres during physical exercise in hot conditions. Sweat glands also respond to emotional stimuli — anxious people perspire more than others.

Sweat has a slightly acrid smell. But this is not particularly heavy in most areas, because sweat provides little in the way of food for the bacteria to thrive. Areas like the feet pose a problem because the sweat becomes trapped by socks and shoes. The heavy odour associated with the armpits is partly because the sweat cannot evaporate easily, and also because there are two other glands (the apocrine glands and the sebaceous glands) at work in this area.

The apocrine glands are also a type of sweat glands, but they have a limited distribution in the armpits, genital area, nipples and eyelids. Apocrine sweat is released in spurts at short intervals. This release is not directly under the control of the nervous system but is dependent on the sex-hormone levels. Even so, the secretions are not just confined to sexual activity and can be triggered off by mental and physical exertion.

Apocrine sweat is odourless when it is produced. It is rich in fats, proteins, and many other organic materials – so it is a rich food for bacteria. The bacteria decompose the sweat to produce the characteristic body odour.

The human apocrine sweat is closely related to the musk that many animals secrete to attract their mates. So whether we realise it or not, apocrine secretions probably act as strong aphrodisiacs – so using deodorants does not necessarily make you more appealing.

The third type of secretory glands are the sebaceous glands. They are distributed all over the body with the exception of the palms and soles; their largest concentration is on the scalp and the face. These glands are also sensitive to hormones and to other stimuli such as stress, anxiety and sexual excitement.

Sebaceous glands secrete an oily lubricant known as sebum which contains cholesterol, fatty acids, waxes and proteins. Sebum, by itself is odourless but it does easily attract bacteria and these can produce strong odours, particularly around the scalp.

The distribution of glands across the body has a great deal to do with how strongly you smell. Some parts like armpits and genitals have a heavy smell because they are richly endowed with all types of glands. Further, these parts are covered, so water cannot evaporate. All these conditions eventually lead to the production of offensive body odours.

Apart from these secretions, the dead skin itself also forms nutritive food for the bacteria. The skin is in a state of continuous change: the old cells at the surface, being replaced by new ones coming from the lower layers. So, there is always a certain amount of dead matter lying on the surface of the body. It is this dead matter which provides additional nutrition for the bacteria.

The bacteria are very pivotal for the production of body odour. There are millions of bacteria living and multiplying on the skin surface. However, much you scrub yourself in the bath, a few million bacteria will survive the onslaught and these then rapidly multiply and colonise the skin again.

Reducing body odour

As mentioned previously, you cannot do much about the bacteria on your skin; any amount of scrubbing or washing would be able to get rid of only fraction of the bacteria and that too for a shortwhile. Neither can you stop yourself from sweating altogether. But there are still several other things that you can do to reduce the amount of sweat you produce:

- Avoid synthetic wear because cotton is definitely cooler than synthetic.

- Also avoid tight fitting clothes, they make the problem of sweating worse.
- Avoid hot drinks and hot crowded places.

The other way to counter body odour is to use products designed to minimise body odours. There are three types of such products available: antiperspirants, deodorants and perfumes. These are available in a variety of forms: lotions, creams, squeeze bottle sprays, roll-ons, pads, aerosol sprays, powders, soap-bars and sticks. Sprays and roll-ons are the most popular formulations.

Antiperspirants contain aluminium salts which reduce the release of sweat by closing the sweat ducts. These are especially useful for people who sweat profusely on the feet.

Deodorants contain an antiseptic to combat bacteria. They do reduce odour but do not cut down the sweating. Therefore, if you have a tendency to sweat a lot, after a few hours the deodorant will be washed away. Most deodorants, in addition, contain perfumes to disguise whatever odours are produced.

●●●

9. Cosmetic Surgery

SCOPE OF COSMETIC SURGERY

Plastic surgery operations were first performed in Egypt and in India, several thousands of years ago. The era of present day plastic surgery, however, began after the First World War – when skins of millions of people had been devastated by burns and scars. Moreover, by then anaesthesia and antiseptics had revolutionised the scope of surgery.

The type of work done by plastic surgeons falls under two main categories:

1. Work done to repair burnt, wounded or distorted tissues – this is known as *reconstructive plastic surgery*.
2. Surgery to make an individual more attractive – this is *cosmetic* or *aesthetic surgery*.

What sort of people require cosmetic surgery?

Several people come to a plastic surgeon wanting changes in their appearance. A good surgeon, however, will consider each case individually, acting as a surgeon, a confidant and a psychiatrist, at the same time.

People who have been involved in accidents or who have sustained burns, can develop scars. Apart from looking ugly, these scars may cause symptoms. In such patients, surgery is not mere vanity but is a necessity – to alleviate the person's symptoms. But many a time, the prime motivation for cosmetic surgery is vanity – here surgery is an extension of the fashion and the beauty industry. Many of these patients do not actually need any surgery, but they have this obsessive desire to look better or even look like a favourite movie star. Several of these people seek cosmetic surgery when they are in the depths of depression – they convince themselves that if they can change the shapes of their nose or have a face-lift, all would be well. It is very much possible that the operation will not live upto these peoples' expectations. The aftermath of surgery then will be a worse depression. An understanding counsellor is probably what they require – and require rather urgently!

If you are contemplating cosmetic surgery, remember the following:

- Consult only a fully qualified and an experienced cosmetic surgeon.
- Decide well in advance exactly what you want changed and to what.

- Do not believe anyone who says that there are no risks involved. Discuss the advantages and disadvantages, frankly with your doctor.
- Talk to someone who has had a similar operation and find out for yourself how he has felt about it.
- Remember that the best of plastic surgeons can, at the best of times, only achieve minor miracles.
- Do not ever over-spend on the surgery — the results are really not worth getting into debts.

COMMON COSMETIC OPERATIONS

For acne scars

Acne scars often cause mental anguish because they tend to be permanent. Scars following acne are of 3 types — the small superficial pits, which are barely visible, the larger pits, which follow inflammed acne and, on rare occasions, the third type of scars may appear — the hypertrophic variety.

Several techniques have been employed to get rid of these scars — the most well-known of these is *dermabrasion* or *sand paper surgery*. This is nothing but removal of the superficial layers of the skin using a rapidly rotating brush. This operation should not be done if active acne is present, because there may be a severe exacerbation.

Dermabrasion has been found useful for treating broad based pitted scars; there is a 50-70% improvement in these scars. One adequate planing gives better results than a number of inadequate surgeries.

The entire face can normally be planed in 15-20 minutes. Slight oozing occurs in the first few hours; the skin then normally heals within a fortnight, after which routine work can be resumed.

For the first few months after surgery, the skin looks pink and there is an increased sensitivity to sunlight. Other complications are usually infrequent, though there might be a slight darkening of the skin.

The second method of reducing scars in acne is using freezing agents like *liquid nitrogen, dry ice,* and *nitrous oxide.* Applications of these agents is followed by redness, scaling and sometimes by blisters. The agent is reapplied after a couple of weeks, till the desired results are obtained. There are several advantages with this method of scar reduction: it is less painful, cheaper and less complicated than dermabrasion; moreover, these agents can be applied even in the presence of active lesions and the results are comparable with those obtained by planing.

Another method of dealing with acne scars is using chemicals like *trichloroacetic acid* and *phenol* to remove the superficial layers of the skin. If not done carefully, this technique can cause superficial burns. But through experienced hands, this technique has given excellent results.

To deal with severely depressed scars, injections of *bovine collagen* are given at the site of the scars. It is yet too early to comment on the value of this rather expensive method of treating acne scars.

Hair transplantation

This operation should be done only if there is no chance of the hair growing back either spontaneously or with medications. There are only few types of baldness for which hair transplantation is resorted to – one of them is male baldness.

Small grafts of hair bearing skin (usually from the back of the scalp) are transferred to bald areas of the scalp. In one sitting, generally about 50-100 grafts can be transplanted. For moderately severe baldness, usually 3-4 sittings are done, at the intervals of 4 weeks. The grafted hairs usually shed within 3 weeks after surgery, but begin to regrow in about 3 months' time.

The final appearance of the person depends to a large extent on good planning and the skill of the surgeon. Infection may occasionally occur and should be vigorously controlled. Rarely scarring occurs – this really ruins the transplant.

CHOOSING YOUR LOOKS

If you are contemplating cosmetic surgery, you may convince yourself that you are going to end up looking like the image of your favourite star – but remember, your surgeon is not going to work from pictures of your favourite star but is going to work on your face. The classical hooked nose may not look quite enchanting on your rather rounded face. So, if you want a particular feature altered, then choose a change which goes with the rest of you and do not stubbornly insist on incongruous changes.

To reshape your face (nose, ears, chin)

A number of changes can be brought about on your face. One of the commonest cosmetic surgeries performed on the face is *rhinoplasty* or the nose repair operation. In experienced and skilled hands, a lot can be done on the nose – a long nose can be shortened, a hump can be removed or a saddle highlighted; a crooked nose can be straightened and a turned-up nose turned down. There are no visible scars because the stitching is done from within. There is, however, one problem: the new nose takes a couple of months to settle down; the area around the nose is swollen and there may be a feeling of stuffiness and numbness, but this gradually disappears.

Ear pinning or *otoplasty* is done for protruding ears. This is a short, simple and completely safe operation. The scar is not visible as the stitches are put behind the ears.

Chin surgery is done either to build the chin up or to cut down its size; a weak chin can be augmented with a silicon mould and a jutting chin can be reduced by removing the excess bone. Surgery can be performed on the cheek bones to highlight them. The final change of appearance following surgery on the chin and on the cheek is dramatic, but there is an initial period of puffiness of the face and this may take a couple of months to subside.

FOR THE WRINKLED SKIN

For the aged and wrinkled skin, a number of operative remedies are available – face lift eye lift, chemical peeling and collagen implants.

Which is the best time for a face lift?

The best time to get a face lift is when you are in the late forties or in the early fifties – though many people have it done before or after. A properly executed face lift can take about ten years off your age. The effect of a face lift is permanent, in that the old wrinkles do not reappear. But since ageing continues, new wrinkles do appear with time. So when age catches up with you again, you can even go for another face lift.

Is there any scarring?

No, there is generally no scarring because the stitches are put in areas, where the scars will either be covered by the hair line or be camouflaged by the natural folds of the skin.

A full face lift deals with deep creases and sagging skin and takes several hours to perform. It is done, usually, under general anaesthesia. Incisions are made along the hair line and behind the ears. The skin is freed from the underlying tissues and is then tightened sufficiently. It is then sewn into its new position and the excess is cut off – the procedure is like removing the surface wrinkles from a piece of cloth by pulling it tight.

Following surgery, the face looks bruised and puffy for a few weeks. Within 3 months, the effects of the surgery become obvious, as the swelling subsides and the scars become inconspicuous. There are, fortunately, only few risks with the face lift. Infection, if it occurs, ruins the procedure. Rarely, the nerve to the facial muscles may be damaged and this could lead to problems. If too much skin is cut off, then the face gets an artificially stretched look, but this rarely happens in experienced hands.

What else can be done for the aged face?

An eye lift is usually part of the full face lift; sometimes this surgery is done alone. The effects are long lasting and the wounds heal quickly. After remaining for a few days in the hospital, one can resume work.

Bags under the eyes can also be removed. This problem is inherited and can make even young people appear tired and old.

Drooping lids can be corrected too and the eyebrows reshaped. A heavily yowled chin or a wrinkled neck can be remedied. Frontal creases can also be removed.

Chemical peeling

A less commonly used technique is to remove the superficial wrinkled skin, using chemicals like *phenol* and *trichloroacetic acid*. Though the results with this are satisfactory, there is always the danger of causing burns.

The other technique is to inject *collagen* into the skin. Earlier plastic surgeons used to inject silicon, but this has been given up as it caused severe reactions in the skin.

CONTOURING THE BODY

Apart from becoming beauty conscious, we are also becoming body conscious – there are today, several procedures available to improve the contour of the body.

Removal of excess fat

This should be done only in exceptional cases. It is definitely better to change your approach to diet and to exercise to get rid of the fat, because after surgery, the fat can well reaccumulate and then you would be back to square one.

In very fat people, a large 'apron' of fat tissue is removed from the abdomen. This operation has aptly been nicknamed *apronectomy*. Body reshaping surgeries can also selectively remove fat from the buttocks, thighs and upper arms.

Can breasts be enlarged?

Yes, and the technique is rather simple. A space is created behind the breast tissue and an artificial breast or prosthesis as it is called, is placed in that space. Some surgeons use even an inflatable prosthesis – but imagine the patient's embarrassment if it deflates. The operation is very simple and takes about 45 minutes. The scars fade with time. The biggest problem with this operation is that the body occasionally reacts to the prosthesis. When this happens, the breasts begin to feel hard and look unnatural. Many suggestions have been forwarded to prevent this reaction from occurring. One is to practise compression exercises after the operation. The other is to manipulate the implant regularly to keep the tissues around it stretched and supple. Once the problem sets in, then it may become necessary to operate and remove the hard tissue.

Breast implants do not increase the risk of cancer, nor can a tumour be missed because of the implant.

Can breasts be reduced in size?

Yes, although the procedure is more time-consuming and complex and it requires hospitalisation of more than a week. To make breasts smaller, the surgeon has to remove some of the breast tissues (mostly fat) plus the skin covering it. The areola and the nipple have then to be repositioned.

Most women are pleased with the final result. The scar is usually not bothersome and there is no problem with breast feeding. A problem which may occur, however, is necrosis of the fat and this may lead to infection. The other problem is that no matter how hard a surgeon tries, both the breasts may not be identical. A few women also complain of decreased sensation of the nipples.

Sagging breasts can be lifted

As a woman grows older, the skin covering the breasts sags. These sagging breasts can be lifted by an operation called *mastopexy*. The skin below the breasts is tightened and the excess removed. The nipples have to be repositioned as the operation not only elevates the breasts, but also makes them smaller. If the patient wants to retain the size of the breasts, a prosthesis is then placed. The scar is small and not visible.

LASER SURGERY

The word 'LASER' stands for Light Amplification by Stimulated Emission of Radiation. Lasers have been used for almost 50 years, to treat a variety of diseases.

Types of lasers

There are several types of lasers which are used for different purposes; and it is not necessary that if a laser is effective in treatment of scars it will be useful for removal of hairs.

Type of laser	Used for
Argon laser	Certain red coloured birth marks Pigmented patches of face To remove tattoos
Dye laser	Red coloured birth marks
Diode laser	Hair removal
Erbium YAG	Skin resurfacing for wrinkles Acne scars

Advantages of laser surgery

- Cosmetic result is good.
- Multiple lesions can be treated.
- Red coloured birthmarks and pigmented lesions can be treated (many of these were earlier considered untreatable).
- Post operative complications are less frequent.

Disadvantages of laser therapy

The treatment is costly since the equipment used is expensive and the operator needs specialised training. A single laser system cannot treat all conditions; therefore more than one type of system is required.

Sometimes scarring, altered skin texture, and local infection complicate laser therapy.

What should you know before you go for laser treatment?

Before you venture into taking laser therapy for a skin disease, it may be appropriate for you to answer the following questions:

- Is laser treatment the most appropriate treatment for your skin condition? It is important to remember that our skin may react in a different way to the laser.
- Is the person, who is going to do the treatment, specialised in laser treatment?
- Is the laser being used appropriate for the treatment of your skin condition? This is very important – a hair removing laser may not be the best for treating birthmarks.
- Are your expectations so high that you think that you will become a Beauty Queen after laser surgery?

●●●

Bibliography

Bennet R : *Fundamental Techniques of Cutaneous Surgery;* Churchill Livingstone, London; 1987.

Burdick KH : *Electrosurgical Apparatuses and their Application in Dermatology;* Thomas Publishers, Spring Field; 1982.

Collins WJN, Forrest JO and Walsh R : *A Handbook for Dental Hygienists;* Wright; Bristol; 1986.

Frost P and Horwitz SN : *Principles of Cosmetics for the Dermatologist;* Mosby CV; St. Louis; 1982.

Moschella SL and Hurley HJ : *Dermatology;* WB Saunders Company, Philadelphia; 1985.

Orfanos CE, Montagna W and Stuttgen G : *Hair Research – Status and Future Aspects;* Springer Verlag, Berlin; 1981.

Khanna N. Dermatology and Sexually Transmitted Diseases. Modern Publishers, New Delhi; 2002.

Tremblay S : *The Professional Skin Care Manual;* Prentice Hall, New Jersey; 1978.

Vwien B : *The Complete Beauty Workshop;* Cavendish Books Ltd., London; 1984.

Whitney EN and Cataldo CB : *Understanding Normal and Clinical Nutrition;* West Publishing Co., St. Paul; 1982.

Be Your Own Beautician

—Parvesh Handa

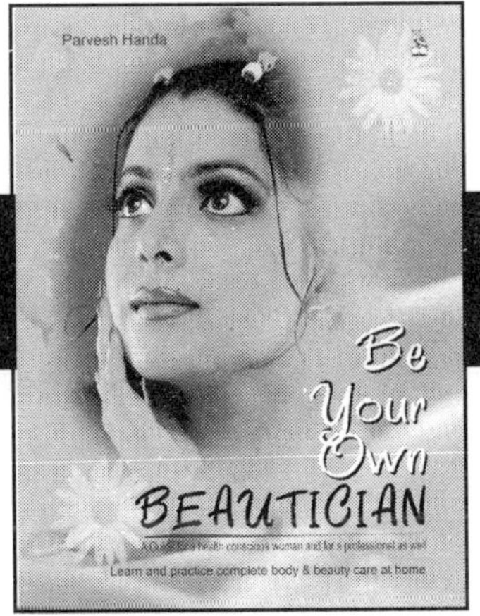

A Guide for a health conscious woman and for a professional as well. Learn and practice complete body & beauty care at home

Those blessed with healthy skin, attractive features, youthful charm and glamorous body are fortunate. This book will tell you exactly how to make and present the best of yourself, how to look radiant from head to feet with the help of natural beauty aids and herbal ingredients. This book describes useful tips for both men and women in detail, to bring out your beauty and explains various questions to the readers:

- If you have chosen the right cosmetics to bring out your beauty?
- How to shape your face, eyes and lips to look their loveliest?
- If you know how to give your type of skin lasting attraction?
- If your hair is alluring and does your hairstyle enhance your personality?
- If you know the secrets of successful figure control?

The author of this book has the honour to write the first book on herbal beauty care published in India in 1982.

Big Size • Pages: 160
Price: Rs. 120/- • Postage: Rs. 20/-